the LA COSTA DIET & EXERCISE BOOK

the LA COSTA

DIET

&

EXERCISE BOOK

R. Philip Smith, M.D.

Publishers · GROSSET & DUNLAP · New York
A FILMWAYS COMPANY

DEDICATION

This book is dedicated to
> M. B. Dalitz
> Allard Roen
> Merv Adelson
> Irwin Molasky

the men who had the vision and the determination to create a complete resort where people can learn a safe, sane way to health, relaxation, and a full enjoyment of their lives.

TABLE OF CONTENTS

PART IV • THE LA COSTA MENU COOKBOOK

ACKNOWLEDGMENTS

The compilation of this book reflects the excellence of the many people on the staff of La Costa who have contributed to its outstanding health program. The La Costa diet and health plan could not have been possible without La Costa, and La Costa could not have been possible if it had not been for the men to whom this book is dedicated.

My deepest gratitude is extended to Mrs. Marjorie Aichele, La Costa's dietitian, who is the backbone of the dining room control. Her excellent knowledge of nutrition and her dedication have done much toward making the La Costa diet a safe and sensible plan.

My thanks also extend to her assistant, Miss Lou Ann Frisch, who has been invaluable in helping put together the food plan for this book and has given much of her time to be of assistance.

No spa in the world has a greater executive chef than La Costa. Chef Willy Hauser's understanding of food and food preparation has truly made low-calorie cooking something a gourmet can appreciate. I owe him my deep gratitude for helping to ensure that the recipes in this book can be used in home kitchens.

Many thanks go to Fred Billak, our first Spa Chef, and to Myles Omel, our present Spa Chef, for their invaluable help and suggestions on preparing low-calorie meals.

The success of the La Costa exercise programs is due to the fine work of Ward Hutton, Director of the Men's Spa, and Doris Hogue, Director of the Women's Spa. Their help has been invaluable in setting forth the innovative and excellent exercise program incorporated in this book. I am especially grateful to Penny Reynolds, an exercise specialist, for her help in the presentation of the exercises and their application.

Many thanks go to Zetta Castle, Director of Public Relations at La Costa. Without her interest and constant encouragement, this book might not have become a reality. I am appreciative of her excellent advice and expertise.

I also thank Beverly Curtis, my secretary, for her fast and accurate typing. Despite the pressures I placed on her, her eagle eye caught numerous errors.

Marion Ortega, R.N., the nurse at the Spa, is due special thanks for helping me to take the time necessary to devote to the manuscript.

Of course, this book would not have been possible if it had not been for the men at Grosset & Dunlap who first approached me with the idea of doing it. Harold Roth, president of Grosset & Dunlap, and Bob Markel, vice-president and editor-in-chief, both felt that the people of America had long been inundated with false information about diets and needed to be led out of the wilderness of unsuccessful and dangerous fads. Both have been most helpful throughout the entire project.

I also thank Jim Neyland for his valuable editorial ability in helping organize the tremendous wealth of material included in this book.

Joyce Frommer has been extremely helpful and friendly with her advice and assistance in editing this book.

I also appreciate the assistance of my two associates, Charles E. Couch, M.D., and Donald B. Jury, M.D., for their critique of the material.

Finally, I must express my gratitude to my wife, Gerry, and to my two children, Bopi and Becky, for tolerating my neglect and for sparing me the considerable time that was necessary to put this book together. Gerry is the literary one in the family, and I could not have done this work without her advice and opinions.

INTRODUCTION

Health spas are not really a new phenomenon. They have existed in Europe and Asia for thousands of years. But La Costa is relatively new. After only twelve years, it has become the world's largest health spa — and for a very good reason: it was set up with a no-nonsense, commonsense approach to nutrition and physical fitness. Collectively, more than 70,000 guests at La Costa have lost over a million pounds in those twelve years. And they have lost that weight with no damage to their health, and with a tremendous sense of acccomplishment, pride, and enjoyment.

In an era of fads and fallacies, that is quite an achievement. But we feel we are just beginning. Even though La Costa is the largest spa in the world, it can accommodate only a certain number of guests at one time. The message that La Costa has to offer should be made available to people everywhere.

That is the purpose of this book: to share with you, the reader, what we have learned and developed to be the safest and most permanent method of weight loss, weight maintenance, and physical fitness available today.

Of course, La Costa is able to pamper its guests with massages, saunas, facials, loofas, herbal wraps, and all the latest available mineral baths and whirlpool baths, and these luxuries cannot be incorporated into a book. But the heart of our program — diet and exercise — is all here in these pages. And there is, literally, something for everyone.

Whatever your age, sex, or physical condition, there are exercises you can perform easily and in the privacy of your home — exercises that will keep you feeling in top form and looking your very best. Even those of you who complain that you have no time for exercise will find that there are movements you can do while you go about your daily activities — in your office, in your kitchen, or even while you bathe or shower. These simple exercises can help you to keep a minimum degree of fitness necessary to function.

If you truly want to keep yourself in top form, I have included a wide variety of exercises you can select from in setting up a daily fourteen-minute program; they include exercises for women, exercises for men, and exercises that two persons can perform together.

But the great value of this program is that it combines diet *and* exercise; it is a complete program for balanced living. This book reveals for the first time La Costa's full fourteen-day menu plan, complete with recipes that you can prepare at home. Just as the guests do at La Costa, you can make selections each day for soups, salads, appetizers, entrées, and desserts, and you will quickly learn an entirely new approach to low-calorie cooking so that you can maintain your weight and health after you have stopped your "diet."

With the La Costa program, you do not have to suffer by denying yourself a long list of favorite foods. You can truly enjoy gourmet meals, with entrées such as Linguini with Clam Sauce, Medallion of Veal Princesse, Lobster Ambassador, Chicken Cacciatore, Beef Stroganoff, and Scampi Provencale You can even have desserts such as Chocolate Mousse, Pumpkin Custard, Coupe St. Jacques, and Buttermilk Sherbet.

Most important, you can tailor both your diet and your exercise program to your own needs, setting your own pace for weight loss, taking into consideration your age, degree of activity, and the amount of weight you truly need to lose. In the process, you will learn much about your own body and about its needs. By utilizing the Dietary Exchange Program, you will never again overeat because of a lack of knowledge — you will know precisely what you are feeding your body and what the effect will be.

If you are overweight, you have probably tried one or more of the "miracle" diets, one of the fads that suddenly sweep the nation and then disappear. This program is not a miracle diet; there are no gimmicks; but its results can truly be "miraculous" if you apply the most important ingredient — *your own intelligence and dedication.*

PART I

BALANCED LIVING

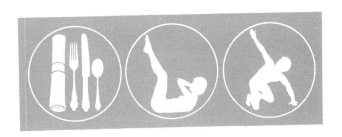

Chapter 1

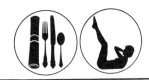

WARNING: THE GOOD LIFE CAN BE DANGEROUS TO YOUR HEALTH

If you are an average American, you are committing a very slow form of suicide. It is called "nutritional roulette," and it is a much more dangerous game than Russian Roulette, because all the chambers except one are loaded. Even though the United States has the best that modern science, medicine, and technology have to offer, it is very difficult to find your way to proper diet and physical fitness amid junk foods, high-fat "gourmet" dinners, chemical additives, fad diets, and the sedentary life style.

Malnutrition in this country has reached alarming proportions — and it is not just the poor who are suffering; it is also the affluent, who have the money to buy whatever foods they want and the time to get the proper exercise, but who choose instead an inadequate diet and a daily routine that encourages physical deterioration.

"Malnutrition" does not mean simply "insufficient food." It refers specifically to the lack of nutrients in the diet and to an improper and inadequate balance to keep the body functioning. Starvation is not the only form of malnutrition. You can be 20 pounds overweight and yet not have the nutrients your body needs to do its job of upkeep.

It has been estimated that six out of every ten people in the United States over the age of twenty-five are overweight. Of those six, three are "overfat," which means that fat tissue has infiltrated the muscular tissue and the tissues of the vital organs. This condition is not always easy to recognize just by looking at a person. Someone may be only 10 percent overweight, while being 20 percent overfat because of inactivity. For example, a man who should weigh 150 might weigh 165 and look presentable; however, he could be 20 percent overfat and endangering his health. Unfortunately, most people do not worry about their diet as long as they maintain a good appearance; they are less concerned with their health than with how they look.

It is interesting to consider how "prime" meat is produced and to compare that process with what we are doing to ourselves. Prime beef is obtained by confining cattle in small pens to keep them from getting exercise and by force-feeding them with a rich high-calorie diet, so that — after they are slaughtered and sold as prime meat — every cut is laced with a fine webbing of fat. If you are overweight, and if you are considerably less active than you ought to be, picture a nice juicy, fat-filled steak as you see it in the supermarket. That is how your own muscles may look if you are the typical American. What you cannot see are the fat deposits under the skin and surrounding the vital organs. It is precisely this combination — overfeeding and underactivity — that we have been practicing on ourselves for too many years.

Fat Is More Than an Ugly Word

Once among the healthiest of the nations of the world, the United States now ranks eighteenth in the life expectancy of men and tenth in the life expectancy of women. Interestingly, statistics show that the nations whose life expectancies are decreasing are those which have all the modern conveniences and an abundance of food.

Although it has been stated and restated in books, newspapers, and magazines that fat is linked to heart disease, stroke, diabetes, hypertension, respiratory ailments, and cancer, the American public has paid little attention.

Perhaps people would be more impressed if they understood the part fat plays in the various diseases. For example, did you know that for every extra pound of fat on your body, your heart has to pump the blood through an extra half-mile of blood vessels? This places an unnecessary strain on your heart, contributes to hypertension, and increases the possibility of coronary occlusion (artery obstruction). Excess fat causes the blood vessels to lose their elasticity; and the inelasticity of the blood vessels contributes toward heart attacks and stroke.

There are two kinds of diabetes — inherited and acquired. Acquired diabetes seems to go along with overweight. Although diabetes is a deficiency disease of the pancreas, it is related to fat because of the instability of the metabolic processes in the body of the overweight person.

Some respiratory ailments are heightened by overweight because the lungs have to work harder to aerate the blood; and the heart has to work harder to force the blood into areas that are not acclimated to take the blood supply.

There has been some medical evidence recently that the deficiency of roughage and fiber in the American diet has increased the incidence of cancer of the colon and rectum. Much of this work was done by Dr. Dennis Burkitt, whose findings have been published in *Lancet*. (Dr. Burkitt is with the Medical Research Council of Great Britain.) An increase of fiber in the diet fundamentally affects the size of the stool, the transit time through the bowel, and the bacterial environment of the bowel. Colon and rectal cancer is most common in the developed nations and lowest in the underdeveloped nations. There is still some question whether it is the lack of fiber in the diet or the high fat content of food that is responsible for the higher incidence of colon and rectal cancer.

Canadian research has shown a connection between fatty, high-calorie diets and breast cancer. At a recent meeting with the National Cancer Institute and the American Cancer Society, Dr. Anthony B. Miller of the National Cancer Institute of Canada announced that ''there appears to be an association between high intake of fat and total calories and breast cancer among women younger than age seventy.'' Dr. Miller also reported: ''The possibility that fat serves as a vehicle for environmental carcinogens must also be considered.''

Cholesterol is, of course, a major problem in our diet. However, many people who have become cholesterol-conscious have the impression that we get all cholesterol directly from eggs and the organ meats. Actually, we get only a small percentage of our total cholesterol in that way. The body manufactures the larger percentage of its cholesterol using fats and some other nutrients. The only way that cholesterol levels can be reduced effectively is by a combination of diet and exercise.

The two main killers of modern man are atherosclerosis and cancer of the lower bowel. Atherosclerosis is characterized by plaques which are laid down as fatty deposits in the vessels of the aorta and the coronary arteries. These plaques are found especially in people who eat too many fatty foods and even appear in children who do not take in the proper type of diet. As the plaques get larger and larger, they contribute to spasm of the vessel. This is the basis of a coronary vascular occlusion, which damages a section of the heart muscle. It is called in lay terms a "heart attack."

By increasing our susceptibility to these degenerative diseases, we are decreasing our life expectancy — both in the number of years and in the enjoyment of those years. If you are overweight and inactive, you should not look upon heart disease, hypertension, stroke, diabetes, respiratory disease, or cancer as something that happens to other people. If you continue to neglect your body, it could happen to you.

OVERFEEDING OURSELVES

The United States has not always been a nation of fat people. Our ancestors may have eaten just as much as we do today, but they needed more nourishment than we do. Most of them worked very hard at physical labor, and they did not have the convenience of automotive transportation, elevators and escalators, gas, electricity, or even running water. In short, they expended a great deal of energy, and therefore needed a great deal of food.

Plumpness, to them, meant good health, because it also meant sufficient nutrients to enable them to fight off infectious diseases, and it meant they had plenty of surplus energy in case they needed it. In the winters, when food was sparse, they had plenty of reserves in fat cells to survive. A good hearty appetite was a sign of health, and they encouraged their families to eat as much as they could, the more the better. "Clean your plate," became an edict from parents to children, generation after generation.

Such edicts were sound, considering the heavily active lives of these early Americans. They were able to build a country while withstanding the infectious diseases to which undernourishment might have exposed them. And, as long as they were active, they did not do severe damage to their bodies by overweight.

These habits have continued into the twentieth century — with serious consequences. Today, we continue to eat like farmers and frontiersmen, while expending considerably less energy than our ancestors did. And we grow more and more "overnourished," becoming more and more susceptible to debilitating diseases. Many of us spend our days sitting in offices or factories, letting machines do the physical labor for us, and then spend our evenings gorging ourselves, letting machines entertain us.

This is presumably what "the good life" is all about; this was the object and the result of all the work and effort of our ancestors. As it was for them, food continues to be the center of our lives; our family, our social gatherings, our entertainment, our holidays — we feel we cannot enjoy these occasions unless we stuff ourselves beyond satiety.

However, simple overeating (membership in the "Clean Plate Club") fills only one chamber of the pistol we use to play nutritional roulette. We cannot blame our ancestors for the four other loaded chambers — inactivity, the snob appeal of gourmet dining, the proliferation of snack foods, and the use of dangerous fad diets.

LACK OF EXERCISE

Inactivity is probably our most serious problem, for which we have no one to blame but ourselves. We may try to excuse ourselves by pointing to the frantic pace of our daily schedules, but we do have some control over that. And the true reason may very well be the opposite — compared with the ease with which we accomplish most things, exercise seems to take too much initiative and energy.

GOURMET DINING

Another problem — one that may not be so readily apparent as a problem — is our recent preoccupation with dining out. The American people have always been enamored of European sophistication. Hence the proliferation of gourmet food shops and gourmet restaurants in the last ten to fifteen years, which has increased our waistbands while increasing our knowledge of world culinary techniques. The rich, fat-filled sauces delight our sense of taste while lush decor and "atmosphere" delight our eyes. For many people, the atmosphere is even more important than the food; as long as the mood is right, they will enjoy themselves no matter what they are eating. The atmosphere and the entertainment disguise the fact that what they are doing is providing their bodies with nutrition. It has reached a point where dining out is the number one form of entertainment in the United States. And the first thing anyone who is traveling does after arriving in a new town and checking into a hotel is to locate the finest local gourmet restaurant.

Admittedly dining out is an enjoyable pastime, and the restaurants themselves are not to blame for our excesses. If we knew how to eat sensibly, we could eat our cake and have it too.

SNACK FOODS

Not only has food become the center of our lives, it has also become big business. Food companies are constantly coming up with new products and advertising them on television in such an appetizing way that we simply cannot resist them — whether they are good for us or not. Fantastic claims are made for these foods, emphasizing catch phrases such as "energy packed," and "high protein," and "sugarless"; and most of us do not know enough about nutrition to distinguish between the claims and the facts. Snack foods have had an enormous impact on our eating (and overeating) habits, adding both unnecessary fat and excessive salt to our diets.

THE FAD DIETS

A considerable number of the overweight people in the United States have been aware of the problems of diet for some time. And these are the people who are also most aware of how the fifth chamber of the gun is loaded, for they have been trying one fashionable ''miracle'' weight-loss diet after another. These fad diets may constitute an even greater danger than the fat they try to remove, because most of them deny the body essential nutrients and substitute starvation for good sense.

If you emphasize one food group and cut out one of the others, you are creating a very serious imbalance in the body. You may very well lose weight for a while (because you are starving the body of nutrients), but you are placing a strain on your system that you will eventually pay for in one way or another.

I recall a patient, an important business executive, who came to La Costa to lose weight after having tried a popular high-protein, low-carbohydrate diet. For the first week on that diet, he had lost weight, but by the second week he was having painful reactions. He was in the third week of his diet when I saw him. His mental faculties had been so severely affected by the diet by that time that he could not remember his own address and phone number. Another patient, a woman on another protein diet, came in to my office having lost 14 pounds in one week but suffering from painful and uncontrollable diarrhea and vomiting. Hospitalization was required to rehabilitate her.

I found it revealing to listen to the proponent of this diet answering questions on a national television show. One woman called in to ask how she could get over a problem she faced with his diet. With each alternative he suggested, she informed him that she had tried it and failed. Finally, his ''solution'' to her problem was ''Well, I guess you just have to bite the bullet'' — hardly a satisfactory response from someone who claims to have a ''miracle'' cure for overweight.

I have in my office more than fifty books, each offering a different method of weight reduction, most of them proclaiming a single food or food group as the magical means. That in itself should make anyone suspicious. In medicine, whenever there are a number of ''cures'' for a specific illness, there is good reason to suspect that none of them is fully effective.

These diets have been correctly labeled ''fad diets.'' They hit the country by storm and last for a short time (long enough for their proponents to collect their profits) and then get discredited, often in the law courts. Although these diets sometimes do produce dramatic weight losses, all too often they cause serious illnesses as well.

From Fatness to Fitness — A Sane Approach

The only safe chamber in playing nutritional roulette is a well-balanced and adequate diet combined with sufficient physical exercise. There is no other way to live and to enjoy a full, healthy life, whether you are at the proper weight or overweight. It *is* possible to lose weight both safely and sensibly with a diet that supplies you with the essential nutrients. And, if you care about your health, it is not only possible, it is necessary.

As a doctor, I had been concerned about the permanent injuries I saw in my patients, injuries that were caused by improper diet and overweight. Usually these problems were not called to my attention until after it was too late. As I saw more and more of my patients suffer from heart attacks, atherosclerosis, hypertension, strokes, and respiratory problems — and saw that most of them had long been overweight and inactive — I began to realize that I could help them more by the practice of preventive medicine. However, since most people do not themselves become concerned until it is too late, it hardly seemed practicable.

When a group of men came to me with the idea of establishing a health spa, I was pleased by the prospect of putting some of my beliefs into practice. They envisioned a resort that would be beautiful and luxurious, yet would also provide the care and education necessary to improve the health and well-being of its guests. Diet and exercise would be an integral part of the spa program.

Twelve years ago, they built La Costa, and I joined them. In those twelve years, La Costa has become the finest and the largest health spa in the world. Countless people have come for sport and relaxation, and for the clear skies and mild weather of Southern California. But more than 70,000 of those who have come to La Costa have come for medical reasons, approximately one-third of them referred by their doctors. While the medical problems have varied, most have been associated with overweight. Most of those 70,000 people have been helped by the La Costa program; none has been harmed by it.

Our first aim has been to restore fitness through proper diet and sensible exercise, our second to educate people so that they will know how to take care of themselves. Our results have been phenomenal; though why anyone should expect anything but positive results from sound nutrition and exercise is beyond me. We have known for a long time what the human body needs for good health, but too many people prefer to ignore the facts and look for a magical diet that promises overnight results.

There is no such thing as instant thinness or instant fitness. It takes time to become obese and to let your muscles atrophy, and it takes time to correct those problems, too. Sound diet and proper exercise should be a way of life, followed constantly; and the earlier in life our children are taught the way, the better off they will be. It has been encouraging to see the increase in the number of young people in their twenties and thirties coming to La Costa in the past few years. These are the people we may truly be able to help by preventing the serious debilitating diseases that might otherwise strike in later years.

Of course, I cannot claim extraordinary success with every patient who has come into my office. Some have given up on the program because they are not sufficiently motivated; the desire for good health and good appearance is not enough. It is unfortunate that some people have to be frightened into correcting their bad habits — either forced into it by their doctors or embarrassed into it by their friends. But all of those who have sincerely wanted to lose weight have succeeded with the La Costa plan.

Motivation does play a great part in achieving normal weight and fitness. There are a multitude of reasons why people get fat, and similarly there are a multitude of excuses why they cannot reduce their weights. I will not even honor some of the excuses I have heard by repeating them; suffice it to say that no excuse is acceptable. You simply must be willing and ready to change your pattern of life.

If you have had difficulty in losing weight, it is very likely that you have a great many bad habits you are not even aware of. For example, you may eat with your eyes rather than with your mouth, overestimating the amount of food that you really need. Or you may not realize how important the appearance of your servings is to your enjoyment of them.

At La Costa, we have been proud of the large number of guests who have lost weight here and who have kept up their motivation to continue losing weight and to maintain a proper weight after returning home. Most people who visit La Costa once come again — either to enjoy the recreational facilities or to continue with their fitness program. Of those who return, more than half weigh less than they did after their first visit. And they generally lost a considerable amount while they were at La Costa. At La Costa, the average weight loss for a man who is 20 percent overweight is approximately 1 to 1½ pounds a day. If a man is 30 percent overweight, his daily weight loss at La Costa may be as high as 2 pounds a day. Women do not lose as rapidly as men; but women at La Costa generally lose between a half and three-quarters of a pound a day.

Women do not lose weight as rapidly as men for a number of reasons. Probably the main reason is that the female system produces the hormone estrogen, which is a "fat binder," and it is difficult for the fat cell to be reduced in size and empty in the presence of large amounts of estrogen. (If you're a woman who has ever been on the Pill, an estrogenic substance, you might have noticed that you gained a few pounds and then had greater than usual difficulty in taking the weight off.) In addition, women do not have the muscle tone to exercise quite as violently as men to burn up calories.

Admittedly, losing weight at the Spa is much easier than losing weight at home, because we do try to help motivate our guests. Unfortunately, most people look upon both diet and exercise as some sort of punishment, so we try to make both very pleasant for them. The meals are elegantly prepared and served in separate courses; this encourages the guests to eat slowly and enjoy one another's company. The exercise program is accompanied by luxurious whirlpools, massages, herbal wraps, loofas, and facials. And no one at the Spa feels he is alone in his efforts to reduce, because there are others all around who are doing the same thing.

You can and should try to do something about helping yourself to enjoy your life while you are on your diet and fitness program. Most of us have been brought up with the feeling that we have to be rewarded for something we do. (Unfortunately, children, like pets, are usually rewarded for their good deeds with something to eat.) Try to treat yourself to things you enjoy while you are dieting — a warm bath, a movie, some new clothes, a massage, a new hairdo — whatever will make you feel good about the important accomplishment.

The secret of La Costa is really no secret at all. It is the most obvious way to good health that there is — sensible eating and sensible exercise. If there is a secret at all, it is in finding the balance of the two and in keeping it as a way of life.

Some of the things that I set forth here — information about fitness and about nutrition — may be things you have heard or read before. But they are things that cannot be repeated too many times, because they are important to your health and well-being. The program itself does take some effort to understand, but it is effort that could very well save your life.

Learning to take care of your body with this program — both internally through the food you eat and externally through exercise — involves learning about nutrition, calories, the Dietary Exchange System used at La Costa, and how to shop and to prepare food. To enable you to use this information to best advantage, I have set forth a specific fourteen-day menu plan, complete with recipes, giving you several choices of foods for each day. The recipes are easy to prepare, and in following them you should begin to see how much food preparation has to do with the excess weight you have been carrying around.

Most important, you are provided with sufficient information about nutrition that you will know what is happening in your own body as you lose weight and improve muscular tone. You should feel better and better each day as you proceed with the program. And, because you will know why your body is responding to what you are doing, the beneficial change that takes place will be much more likely to be a permanent one. That beneficial change is something we call fitness.

Chapter 2

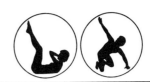

FITNESS

A great many of the guests who come into my office at La Costa are successful business people, men and women with exceptional minds, perceptions, and abilities. I am amazed to find that so many of them have allowed their bodies to deteriorate to the point — for example — where they cannot even take the few steps up to their rooms without losing their breath completely. These men and women, constantly active with their minds, are so inactive physically that they are prime candidates for serious diseases.

Fitness and health are not precisely the same thing, but the two do go hand in hand. Being healthy means being free of disease. A man or woman can be healthy without being fit; he or she can be well nourished, can have a good heart, good eyesight, good hearing, no gastrointestinal problems. But that condition of health might not last for long without fitness.

Physical fitness is the condition of the body that makes people feel and look good, and have enough energy and enough physical reserve to enjoy life. That includes both the ability to do their work all day and the reserve to go home and play some tennis or go swimming, or work in the garden, or play with the children. Anyone who is physically fit should feel able to do whatever he or she wants and not get sluggish and tired. He or she should certainly have enough reserve to meet an emergency, such as having to make a sudden dash across the street to keep from getting hit by a car.

There are actually two different kinds of fitness. If someone is free of disease, I would say that he or she is *organically* fit. A person who is organically fit has practically no infirmities, is well nourished, and can get up and go to work every day. His teeth are all right; his eyes are all right; he is in good general health.

However, there is another kind of fitness, which I call *dynamic* fitness, that is essential to maintaining organic fitness. Dynamic fitness might be defined as the ability to move. Without it, a man or woman is sluggish, cannot climb stairs or run for a bus without getting out of breath; he or she simply lacks endurance. The muscles have begun to atrophy and the respiratory system and the cardiovascular system may be weak.

Most young people and children stay relatively fit; the loss of dynamic fitness generally occurs somewhere in adulthood. After an active youth, most people today settle into sedentary lives. And the more they settle, the less fit they become.

This can be seen clearly in the case of an athlete who quits after having been very active in college or perhaps as a professional. If he continues to eat an athlete's diet and neglects exercise, he soon begins to deteriorate, picking up 50 to 60 pounds in the first year of inactivity. The same thing happens in a lesser way with older people as they spend more and more time in their offices, becoming fatigued from the work of the day and unable to find the time to exercise. They may develop a large bank account, but they also develop a large abdomen, and their muscle tone becomes poor.

The problem in each case is a lack of balance between intake of food and expenditure of physical energy through exercise.

Exercise versus Activity

Many times I have heard patients say, "Why, I get plenty of exercise; I go out and play golf at least twice a week." Sometimes it is difficult to convince them that golf is not an exercise but an activity. Considering the way most people play golf, they would get much more exercise by going for a good brisk walk. Golfers today rarely ever walk the course; they ride in a little motorized cart; and they never carry their own clubs.

Of all the outdoor sports, golf probably burns up the fewest calories, and it is probably also the least effective as exercise for general fitness. However, no single sport could be considered adequate exercise for the entire body. Most professional and college athletes realize this, and they always include general conditioning exercises in their regimen.

Some people have the impression that they can get all the exercise they need from jogging. Jogging can be good for the legs, thighs, the cardiovascular and respiratory systems, but it does little for the rest of the body. And for burning up calories and helping to lose weight it is only slightly better than a good brisk walk. It is interesting to note that the same number of calories are burned up in a person who jogs a mile as in a person of the same weight who walks a mile. The jogger may do it in eight minutes and the walker may take twenty minutes, but the same number of calories are burned up.

Activities such as golf, tennis, and jogging should be looked on as something you do for pleasure, not as your way of getting the exercise your body needs. If you are going to consider activities and exercise as connected at all, you should look upon exercise as something you do so that you will get more pleasure out of your activities.

Exercising the Heart

One of the most important things that exercise does is to raise your pulse. I feel it is extremely important to everyone to get his or her pulse rate up to 120 beats per minute at least once a day, for a period of one to three minutes. It is the only way that you can effectively exercise the muscle that is your heart; it places an extra load on the cardiovascular system, makes the heart work harder, and gives it a chance to develop its musculature.

The heart is a muscular organ with vessels and nerves. When a coronary artery becomes unable to carry blood to a corresponding portion of the heart muscle, we call this condition a coronary occlusion. A section of the muscle of the heart is badly damaged. After the acute phase passes and this section begins to heal, the only way to rehabilitate the heart muscle is to exercise it — and that means putting a load on the heart and making it beat faster. Many patients are sent to La Costa at this stage of their rehabilitation by their cardiologists for a careful program of increasing exercise which includes walking and light physical exertion. We feel that if this exercise program is good for the heart once it is damaged, it certainly is a good program to institute to prevent a heart attack.

The effect of exercise on the heart is that the heart becomes stronger. There is much less chance for vascular insult because the muscles of the heart are pumping more and more blood to the various areas of the organ. The elasticity of the vessels does not deteriorate and the circulation is much improved.

If you do not already know how, you should learn to take your pulse. You will need a watch with a sweep second hand. (1) Place the watch in your left hand with the palm up. (2) Place your left wrist over the right wrist (palm up) so that you can curve the fingers of your right hand to the upper portion of the left wrist. (3) Let the fingers of the right hand gently touch the base of the thumb and slide into the notch just below that. Here you will find the pulse as long as you are not pressing too firmly. (4) Count the pulse rate for 30 seconds and multiply by two.

The normal pulse rate varies but is generally found to be somewhere between 70 and 80 beats per minute. When taking the pulse after exercise, do it as soon as possible after stopping the exercise. Then rest for three minutes and take the pulse again. The rate should slow down by approximately 20 beats.

Flexibility

Agility is a very important part of youth, and we do not want to lose this as we get older. At La Costa we use exercise so that people can enjoy their favorite sports and can move more freely and safely, without losing their balance, which is a problem that often develops with age. No one in his or her sixties or seventies should have to shuffle. There is no reason that older people should not be able to walk briskly and in an erect position.

Muscles develop only if they are exercised; if they are not, they become soft and flabby, losing tone and elasticity. Usually we do not see any need to improve strength and endurance as we get older; but the more strength and endurance we can add to a muscle, the better it is going to perform.

In this respect, the human body is much like an automobile. If you let a car sit in the garage for a year or two, the "joints" (or the mechanical parts of the car) get stiff. This is what happens to a human being who goes for a long period without exercising. Proper exercise stretches muscles, improves the motion of joints, and gives the body flexibility.

Levels of Exercise — Degrees of Fitness

The trouble with most exercise programs is that they seem to be too difficult for the average person to accomplish. Fitness programs are usually created by athletes, and the books on the subject of fitness and exercise are very often written by very athletic people. The average person, however, should not feel that he or she has to compete with anybody, especially with a physical education specialist. It is simply not necessary to be able to do as much as he can do, to be able, say, to do 100 sit-ups or to lift 120 pounds forty times. Each person has his or her own level for maintaining alertness, quickness, and mobility.

Exercise can be directed toward accomplishing several different ends, each of them important in its own way. It is important for the individual to decide which end he or she has in mind, because it will determine how the exercises are performed and, in some cases, which exercises as well.

Of course, each person who comes to me and to La Costa comes with a slightly different physical problem or set of problems. A new mother might come to get back into shape after giving birth; someone else might be at the right weight but want to tone up a few flabby spots; an athlete might want to go into intensive training. At the extreme, there might be someone weighing over 300 pounds needing to lose a great many pounds over many months, or a severely ill person sent by his doctor to get his cardiovascular system sufficiently strong to be able to survive an operation.

Each person, with the help of his or her physician, must determine the degree of fitness he or she needs or wants. While the specific needs may vary, I find that there are four general levels of exercise for four different degrees of fitness. At the first level, one is merely trying to maintain the minimum degree of fitness required to keep fairly active and enjoying life. This bare minimum is accomplished with little exercise — nothing more than a few bending and stretching exercises, and a few isometrics and isotonics.

The second degree of fitness is for those who want to have a little more than the sedentary life — who want to be able to play an occasional game of tennis or golf, or want to be able to mow the lawn once in awhile, or perhaps swing the kids or grandkids up in the air when they greet them. This second level of exercise requires a few real exercises, but nothing really strenuous or taxing.

The third level is what I would consider an athletic level, where one does specific exercises for specific parts of the body to develop the strength and endurance for considerable physical exertion. There are not too many people who want this degree of fitness, and there are not too many who really need it.

The fourth level of exercise is something quite apart from the other three, and it is perhaps the most important. This is the level necessary for weight loss. Unlike the other levels, where the object is to tone and firm and build what one already has, the object of this kind of exercise is to lose. And the only way to lose is to burn up calories. There are about 3500 calories in a pound of fat; to lose one pound a week, a man or woman has to burn up 500 more calories a day than he or she is taking in. This can be done by cutting down on the number of calories taken in, or by increasing exercise to burn up more, or by a combination of both. (Of course, there is a limit to the number of pounds an individual can lose rapidly. Since this depends on the general health and amount of excess weight a person has, I will leave that piece of advice up to your physician.)

It is this combination that I have found to have the most effective and the most lasting results in weight loss. However, there is one further ingredient I consider to be essential for losing weight without gaining it back two weeks later — and that is proper nutrition.

DETERMINING YOUR EXERCISE LEVEL

Some level of exercise is essential for all of us, even if it is just the least amount needed to keep our respiratory and cardiovascular systems operating freely. But there are a great many ways to exercise, and a variety of levels to choose from. The level you choose depends entirely upon how you want to look and feel.

Many people wrongly assume that they get plenty of exercise, because they feel fatigued at the end of the day. Often they feel fatigued in the mornings as well, after a good night's sleep. This is more likely to be so if you have *not* been getting the proper exercise. Generally, the more you exercise, the better you will feel.

Beyond what I consider the minimum daily requirement of exercise, there are two basic objectives you can set for yourself. The first, and the simplest, is to tone and firm your body at its present weight. The second is to expend energy and to lose weight. You can use the same sets of exercises for both objectives. The major difference is that for toning and firming, you exercise slowly; and for weight loss, you perform the exercises as rapidly and as strenuously as you can.

However, do not set out to tone and firm your body at its present weight, and then change your mind and decide to exercise for weight loss. Once you have firmed your body at one weight, it may be difficult to slim down. If losing weight is your first objective, save the toning and firming for later.

You may choose, of course, to lose all the weight you need to lose through exercise. However, if you are severely overweight, it may take you some time. And you may have some difficulty figuring precisely how much energy you spend in your daily activities and how much more energy you must spend to reduce. The table on page 17 gives you the energy cost of activities per hour per pound so you can determine approximately how many calories you use up each day; then you can figure out how you can spend more. We do burn up calories no matter what we are doing, even while sleeping.

It may simplify your calculations to divide these activities into four general types, and then average them out over your day. The first category consists of very light, common activities such as dressing, driving a car, eating, doing laundry, and standing, which burn up less than one calorie per pound of body weight per hour.

The second category is light activity, including dancing, bicycling, making beds, ironing, and playing a musical instrument. These burn up more than one calorie per pound of body weight per hour.

The third category is moderate activity, such as playing table tennis, skating, sweeping with a vacuum cleaner, walking rapidly, and playing tennis. They burn up between 2 and 3 calories per pound of body weight per hour.

The heavy activities that make up the last category are those which burn up more than 2 calories (and sometimes a good deal more) per pound of body weight per hour. These include football and fencing, walking at a high speed, rowing, skiing, and, of course, severe exercise.

Most of our daily activities belong to categories one and two. Seldom do we get into the third category and very seldom into the fourth unless we are attempting to lose weight or to get into condition rapidly.

To try to figure out how many calories you burn during the day, you will have to do quite a bit of arithmetic, and you will have to estimate the number of hours — or fragments of hours — you spend in each activity.

Remember that a pound of fat is about 3500 calories, and to lose one pound a week, you will have to burn up 500 extra calories a day. For example, if you weigh 150 pounds and you want to lose a pound a week, you would have to exercise in the severe (3 calories per pound per hour) to very severe (4 calories per pound per hour) category a full hour each day to reach that goal. At the severe exercise level, the 150-pound person would burn approximately 450 calories in one hour's time. At the very severe exercise level, he or she would burn approximately 600 calories in an hour.

As I have indicated before, I recommend a combination of diet and exercise for losing weight. If you can afford to spend an hour a day in exercise, you are that much further ahead in the game; but ten to fifteen minutes a day is just about as much time as the average person can spend on exercise.

It is also important to realize that if you have been inactive for a long time, you must start your exercise program slowly, or at a moderate speed. If you try to start off with a full hour of vigorous exercise the first day, your program may not last to the next day, because you will be too sore to move. Your object, presumably, is to get fit and to stay fit. If you have a lot of weight to lose before you can become fit, you may want to devote between fifteen and thirty minutes to good solid exercise. However, once you have reached your proper weight and fitness, I recommend a continuing exercise program of under fifteen minutes a day just to keep limber, loose, and properly toned.

When you have reached your proper balance of calorie consumption and calorie expenditure, you will know it because you will feel great. That is the time to make a vow to stick to sensible eating habits and a sensible daily exercise program.

FITNESS IS NOT ALWAYS THINNESS

In trying to determine if you are overweight, you should try to look at yourself objectively. Fit people do not necessarily have to look like fashion models or football players. Research into body types has shown that we are not all built the same way. About thirty years ago, Dr. William H. Sheldon made a survey and found that people fell generally into three basic body types. He called his technique ''somatotyping,'' or ''body typing.''

THE ENERGY COST OF ACTIVITIES

Activity	Calories per pound per hour	Activity	Calories per pound per hour
Bedmaking	1.9	Piano playing (Mendelssohn's "Song Without Words")	0.9
Bicycling (Centry run)	4.0	Piano playing (Beethoven's "Appassionata")	1.1
Bicycling (moderate speed)	1.6	Piano playing (Liszt's "Tarantella")	1.4
Boxing	5.7	Reading aloud	0.7
Carpentry (heavy)	1.5	Rowing	5.0
Cello playing	1.1	Rowing in race	7.8
Cleaning windows	1.7	Running	3.7
Crocheting	0.7	Sawing wood	3.1
Dancing, moderately active	2.2	Sewing, hand	0.7
Dancing rhumba	2.8	Sewing, foot-driven machine	0.8
Dancing waltz	1.9	Sewing, electric machine	0.7
Dishwashing	0.9	Singing in loud voice	0.9
Dressing and undressing	0.8	Sitting quietly	0.7
Driving car	0.9	Skating	2.1
Eating	0.7	Skiing (moderate speed)	5.2
Exercise		Standing at attention	0.8
very light	0.9	Standing relaxed	0.7
light	1.1	Sweeping with broom, bare floor	1.1
moderate	1.9	Sweeping with carpet sweeper	1.2
severe	3.0	Sweeping with vacuum sweeper	2.2
very severe	4.0	Swimming (2 mi. per hr.)	4.1
Fencing	3.8	Tailoring	0.9
Football	3.6	Tennis	2.8
Gardening, weeding	2.3	Typing, rapidly	1.0
Golf	1.2	Typing, electric typewriter	0.7
Horseback riding, walk	1.1	Violin playing	0.8
Horseback riding, trot	2.5	Walking (3 mi. per hr.)	1.4
Horseback riding, gallop	3.5	Walking rapidly (4 mi. per hr.)	2.0
Ironing (5-lb. iron)	1.0	Walking at high speed (5.3 mi. per hr.)	4.3
Knitting sweater	0.8	Walking down stairs, calories per pound per 15 steps	0.011
Laboratory work	1.5		
Laundry, light	0.6	Walking upstairs, calories per pound per 15 steps	0.034
Lying still, awake	0.5		
Office work, standing	0.8	Washing floors	1.0
Organ playing (1/3 handwork)	1.2	Writing	0.7
Painting furniture	1.2		
Paring potatoes	0.8		
Playing cards	0.7		
Playing table tennis	2.5		

(Adapted from Foundations of Nutrition, 6th ed. by Clara Mae Taylor and Oreca Florence Pye. Copyright © 1966, The Macmillan Company.)

There is one group of thin, nervous types, whom he called ectomorphs. These are the people who are models, high jumpers, and such. They have long fingers and long bones. They rarely have a weight problem, unless it is under-weight.

The middle group consists of stocky, muscular types whom he called mesomorphs. They are the people who like bodily exercise, who go for sports and physical education.

The third group he called endomorphs. They are people who are chubby or plump, who love comfort, ease, and the pleasures of the senses.

Someone who is truly an endomorph simply cannot expect to look like a fashion model, nor should someone who is an ectomorph expect to have a round face. To be perfectly fit, you have to be yourself. If, with reasonable diet and exercise, you feel that you *look* chubby, you may be an endomorph. The more important consideration is *how you feel*.

Of course, you will feel your best when your body has found the proper balance of energy output with food consumption — the right amount of exercise combined with good nutrition. This latter is not a subject to be dismissed lightly, especially today, when it is so easy to follow food fads rather than common sense.

Chapter 3

NUTRITION

The food that you eat keeps you alive, makes it possible for you to breathe, for your heart to beat, for you to grow, and for you to have the energy you need to work and play. Most people do know that much, but the average American knows almost nothing about nutrition. Food is what you eat; nutrition is how your body uses the food; and the specific elements within the food that it uses are called nutrients.

Nutrients are essential for growth, for building up the body tissues, for keeping them up, and for replacing worn-out parts. They are needed throughout life, but the amounts of each may vary at different times and with different people. Larger amounts of nutrients are required for body growth when we are young, but some amount of all of them are still required as we grow older. Generally, males need a larger amount than females do; and big people require more than smaller people. Active people require more than do people who are inactive. When we are ill, the nutrients are more important to us than when we are healthy. If a diet lacks nutrients for a long period of time, the body may try to compensate in some way. A good example of this is the absorption of calcium in the body. Calcium is needed in developing bones, making nerves and muscles function, and aiding in the clotting of blood. If the body does not receive enough calcium in the food that is eaten, it must get it from somewhere, so it steals calcium from the bones. If this borrowed calcium is not replaced, it can cause serious damage.

Nutrients are able to work singly and in combination with each other. For example, calcium builds strong bones, but if vitamin D is not present, the calcium is not absorbed and the bone formation does not progress. Protein is a dynamic, important nutrient, but in order for protein to be burned properly and with maximum efficiency, carbohydrate must be present.

The Basic Nutrients

There are six basic nutrients the body needs to *survive*. (There are about forty to fifty nutrients essential to *good health*.) They are water, protein, carbohydrate, fat, minerals, and vitamins. They are all essential to the healthy human body; and none of them can be left out entirely for very long without serious consequences.

WATER

Water ranks next to air or oxygen in importance as an ingredient for life. Between one-half and two-thirds of the body is made up of water. It is much more important to the body than food. You can live for days or weeks without food, but you can survive only a few days without water. There are no calories in water, but still it is an essential nutrient.

Water is necessary for body fluids, and for secretions and excretions. One of its major functions is to carry food materials from one part of the body to the other. Even digestion is dependent upon fluid; all nutrients are dissolved in water so that they can be absorbed in the intestinal tract, and water is very important in the regulation of body temperature as well.

The most significant source of this vital nutrient is the water that a person drinks, but the body does get some fluids as well from fruits and vegetables, milk, coffee, and tea. When food is burned in the body to transform it into energy, a certain amount of water is produced.

PROTEIN

After water and fat, protein is the most plentiful nutrient in the body. It is interesting to note that the body's percentage of fat and protein changes as one gets older. At the age of twenty-five, 15 percent of the body is fat and 14½ percent is protein. At the age of forty-six, 19½ percent of the body is fat while 18½ percent is protein. Protein is required for life itself. It is the dynamic builder of body tissue, and it is the basic ingredient of every cell in the body. Protein is necessary to make hemoglobin, an ingredient of the blood that carries oxygen to the cells and carries carbon dioxide away. The antibodies that the body uses to resist and fight infection are also made up of protein. Protein may supply energy in the absence of carbohydrate. This is a wasteful procedure.

After we eat our food, our bodies break protein down into smaller units, called amino acids, which the body uses in a multitude of ways — some to replace dead cells, some to repair wounds, some to produce new hair and skin, some to develop antibodies. The list of work done by amino acids is endless.

The body can make its own supply of about half of the amino acids, but the others must come directly from the foods taken into the body. The foods that supply the largest number of amino acids are those from animals, such as beef, pork, lamb, fish, poultry, eggs, and milk. The proteins from cereals, vegetables, fruits, and nuts do not provide as complete an assortment of amino acids as the animal proteins, but they can be a valuable source of some of them. Some vegetables — such as soybeans, legumes, and peanuts — are almost as good a source of protein as the animal sources.

If your body does not get sufficient protein, you become susceptible to a multitude of ailments — from blood diseases to problems with bones, muscles, and internal organs. If the body gets excess protein (it can use only a certain amount at one time), it converts the excess into fats. If insufficient carbohydrate is present, it can be formed from protein, but this procedure is wasteful and overworks the liver and kidneys. Fifty-eight percent of the protein ingested is converted to carbohydrate when no carbohydrate is ingested in the regular diet.

CARBOHYDRATE

Carbohydrate is the major source of energy in the diet. It is found primarily in three forms — starches, sugars, and celluloses. Starches and sugars are sources of energy, while cellulose furnishes bulk in the diet. In supplying energy, carbohydrate helps to save the protein for tissue building and repair, and for other special jobs. Carbohydrate is also an aid in the metabolism of protein.

The form of carbohydrate found mostly in vegetables is starch. The best sources of starch are the grains, such as wheat, oats, corn, and rice, from which are made flour, macaroni, spaghetti, noodles, breads, and cereals. Potatoes, sweet potatoes, dried beans, and peas are also good sources of starch. Starches are important for energy reserve, because they can be stored in the liver and muscles as glycogen for use when needed.

In fruits and fruit juices, carbohydrate is found in the form of sugars. Some of the concentrated sources of sugar are cane and beet sugars, jellies, jams, candy, honey, molasses, and syrups. Carbohydrates are absorbed as glucose, which is the principal supplier of energy for the entire body.

Carbohydrate is essential to the proper functioning of the nervous system and the brain, as well as important in the functioning of muscles and organs. If you do not get enough carbohydrate (as in the case of some reducing diets), the brain ceases to function properly, you become forgetful or absent-minded, and you can become depressed. Another thing that happens with insufficient carbohydrate is that the body has to convert some of its valuable protein to carbohydrate through a process called glyconeogenesis, and this places a considerable strain on the liver and kidneys.

If you eat an excess of carbohydrate, it is stored in the body as fat.

FAT

Fat is indeed a necessary part of the nutrition of the body. It forms a part of each cell in the body, and it protects and cushions the vital organs. In a cold climate, fat can also be an aid in controlling body warmth by serving as insulation against heat loss.

Fats are a highly concentrated source of energy; they give you 2¼ times the amount of energy or calories as do the carbohydrates and proteins in like amounts. Fats and carbohydrates help the body to conserve protein for building and repairing itself by furnishing energy so that the protein will not have to be used for this purpose.

While the principal use of fat in the body is to produce and supply energy, fats also serve the important function of carrying the fat-soluble vitamins A, D, E, and K.

One important fatty acid the body needs but cannot produce is linoleic acid. It must be obtained through food. It is found in good quality and amount in the polyunsaturated fats — in margarines, salad dressings, mayonnaise, and nonhydrogenated cooking oils. Poultry and fish also have considerable linoleic acid. Because of the importance of linoleic acid, you must include a certain amount of the polyunsaturated fats in your diet.

Fats are popular foods because they add flavor, texture, eye appeal, and satiety to the diet. Fats exclude air, so they prevent the drying of meats and vegetables. Because they remain in the stomach longer, and the body metabolizes them more slowly than it does carbohydrates, the feeling of hunger does not return quite so rapidly after eating them.

The best sources of fat are margarine, butter, salad oil, cream, cheese, mayonnaise, salad dressings, nuts, and bacon and other fatty meats. Some natural fat is also found in meats, whole milk, eggs, chocolate, and avocado.

Because of the close relationship between cholesterol and heart attacks, most Americans today are very conscious of their cholesterol count. Cholesterol is a fatlike substance that is found in every cell in the body. Approximately 60 percent of the cholesterol in our bodies is manufactured by the body itself, while the remaining 40 percent is obtained from the food we eat. When attempting to control a high cholesterol count, eating foods that are low in cholesterol, and avoiding those that are high, can aid in lowering the cholesterol level in the bloodstream. However, in my experience, a major factor in lowering cholesterol blood levels is an increase in exercise. Burning up the cholesterol by the use of exercise is often more effective than trying to control it by diet alone.

The largest amounts of cholesterol in foods are in the organ meats of animals (such as brains, liver, and kidney) and egg yolk, although some quantity is supplied by shellfish. Other types of fish, poultry, and lean meats contain only small amounts of cholesterol.

MINERALS

A number of mineral elements are vital to the proper functioning of the body — such minerals as calcium, iron, iodine, zinc, copper, sodium, potassium, magnesium, and phosphorus. Some of them are found in fairly large amounts in the body, but others are considered only trace minerals, those of which a small amount supplies the needs of the body. Minerals help to give strength and rigidity to the tissues, and they also assist the functioning of the organs, muscles, and nerves and aid in the clotting of blood.

Calcium: The most abundant mineral element in the body is calcium. Combined with phosphorus, it is responsible for the hardness of bones and teeth. It has been estimated that 99 percent of the calcium in the body is found in these two tissues. Calcium is necessary to the clotting of blood, and it has a great deal to do with the conduction system in the heart. Nerve tissue is also dependent on the calcium level in the blood.

Milk is our best source of calcium, and for this reason all well-balanced dietary regimes include milk. Two cups of milk (or its equivalent in cheese) will supply most of the calcium we need each day. Dark green leafy vegetables also provide some calcium, and salmon and sardines are a good source as long as the tiny bones are eaten.

Iron: Iron is an essential mineral. It combines with protein to make hemoglobin, and it also helps the cells to obtain their necessary energy from foods. We can get about 25 percent of our daily requirement of iron from whole-grain and enriched bread and cereal. The rest of it must be obtained from lean meats, shellfish, dried beans and peas, dried fruits, egg yolk, and molasses.

Women require more iron because of the loss of blood during menstruation.

Iron deficiency diseases are especially common in children, teenagers, and women in pregnancy (because of the demands of the fetus).

Iodine: An insufficient amount of iodine in one's diet can cause a deficiency disease called goiter, which is an enlargement of the thyroid gland. It is found most often away from the seacoast, where food is grown in soil deficient in this mineral. Sufficient iodine can be obtained by occasional inclusion of seafood in the diet, and by the proper use of iodized salt.

Sodium will be discussed at length in Chapter 4 on "Salt and Sugar in Weight Control."

VITAMINS

Vitamins are chemicals that aid in releasing energy from foods and in stimulating chemical reactions. They promote the normal growth of different kinds of tissue; they are essential for the proper functioning of nerves and muscles; and they facilitate the utilization of foods. Vitamins are found naturally in the foods we eat, and if we eat a balanced diet of foods that have been prepared properly, we do not need vitamin supplements in the form of pills. In recent years, the public has been bombarded by books and advertising claiming miraculous curative powers for massive doses of certain vitamins. Most of these claims have not been substantiated through research. It has been proved, however, that excessive or prolonged use of some of these vitamins can cause serious medical problems.

If, for some reason, your diet is imbalanced, a multivitamin from a reputable national drug company is all that you need. I advise you to avoid purchasing locally prepared and packaged vitamins in so-called health food stores, because you have no assurance of getting exactly what you are paying for. Since they are not sold interstate, these vitamins are not regulated by the Food and Drug Administration.

Vitamin A: Vitamin A is necessary for normal growth. It is important in the function of the eye, aiding in normal vision, especially in dim light, and lack of this vitamin can cause a condition known as "night blindness." Vitamin A also helps the skin and the mucous membranes to resist infection.

Vitamin A is found only in foods of animal origin, but fruits and vegetables that are deep yellow or dark green contain a material called carotene, which the body can convert into vitamin A. Liver is the most important source of vitamin A; a 2-ounce serving of cooked beef liver can provide approximately six times more than the individual requires in one day. Margarine and whole milk and milk products such as cheese are also good sources. However, skim milk has no vitamin A, unless it is "fortified" skim milk, which has vitamins A and D added.

There is sufficient vitamin A in fruits and vegetables such as dark greens, carrots, squash, sweet potatoes, yellow peaches, cantaloupe, and papaya to take care of one's daily requirement. Unless there is a medical reason determined by a doctor, there is no need for anyone to take supplements of vitamin A.

Excessive intake of vitamin A for a prolonged period can cause pressures within the head resembling the pains caused by brain tumors. Also, people who consume tremendous amounts of carrot juice, which is rich in carotene, develop a condition called carotenemia, which causes the skin to turn yellow.

Vitamin B: There are a number of B vitamins, and they are all important in the body for the release of energy from food. They have a great deal to do with the functioning of the nervous system; they aid in keeping the digestive system functioning calmly; and they help to maintain a healthy skin. Some of the most important B vitamins are vitamin B_1 (called thiamine), vitamin B_2 (called riboflavin), niacin, vitamin B_6, and vitamin B_{12}.

Lean pork is the most common source of B_1, although it is also found in dried beans and peas, in some of the organ meats, and in nuts. A smaller source is whole-grain and enriched cereals, rice, breads, and yeast. Lack of vitamin B_1 causes a disease known as beriberi, which is occasionally associated with severe alcoholism.

Vitamin B_2 is found in plentiful supply in meats, milk, and whole-grain and enriched breads and cereals. Organ meats, especially liver and kidney, also produce some of this vitamin.

Niacin is found in meat and meat products, and in whole-grain and enriched cereals. Peas and beans also have some niacin. The body has the ability to turn one of its essential amino acids, tryptophan, into niacin.

Vitamin B_6, vitamin B_{12}, and folacin (or folic acid) are necessary for the manufacture and maintenance of the hemoglobin in the bloodstream, and they are of considerable importance in preventing anemia. These vitamins are found mostly in foods of animal origin. Strict vegetarians often develop a B_{12} deficiency, which shows up as a soreness of the mouth and tongue, accompanied by numbness and tingling of the hands and legs, and is often accompanied by a severe loss of coordination.

Vitamin C: Vitamin C is ascorbic acid, and it is found in plentiful supply in many foods. Citrus fruits such as oranges, grapefruits, tangerines, and lemons are especially rich in C. Fresh strawberries and vegetables such as tomatoes, cabbage, green peppers, spinach, and potatoes and sweet potatoes also contain much vitamin C.

Vitamin C helps the body to maintain the cementing material called collagen that holds the cells together, and it aids in strengthening the walls of the blood vessels. It also helps in the prevention of tooth decay and pyorrhea.

Although it has been highly touted as a preventer of colds, this has never been conclusively proved by medical research. Excessive doses of vitamin C can cause diarrhea; and in Russia large doses of the vitamin C have been used to induce early abortion.

Vitamin D: Vitamin D is often referred to as the sunshine vitamin because our bodies are able to produce it if the skin is exposed to direct sunlight. Without vitamin D, the body cannot absorb the calcium that is supplied in the food we eat. For that reason, vitamin D is extremely important during early growth for the building of strong bones and teeth. Although adults seldom need more vitamin D than they normally obtain from their food or from the sun, tiny infants and young children may not get the necessary amount. If they do not, they develop a disease known as rickets because they have absorbed too little calcium. The bones of a child with rickets are soft, and so he or she often has deformed legs, enlarged joints, knock-knees, and occasionally beaded ribs (a series of visible prominences at the points where the ribs join their cartilages).

Few foods naturally contain vitamin D. Supplements such as cod liver oil and halibut liver oil plus sunshine can be prescribed. However, milk is usually fortified with vitamin D.

Taken in excessive and prolonged doses, vitamin D can be extremely dangerous, overloading the blood and the body tissues with calcium and causing calcification in the soft tissues. Bone deformities can develop in both adults and children. There have been numerous reports of children developing calcium deposits in the kidneys and some of the other organs, resulting in permanent damage. There have also been reports of vitamin D toxicity, with serious consequences.

Because of these dangers, the Food and Drug Administration restricts the dosage of over-the-counter vitamin D to 400 units and of vitamin A to 10,000 units. Larger dosages of these vitamins cannot be purchased unless prescribed by a physician.

Vitamin E: The sudden popularity of vitamin E as a cure-all is astonishing. The claims for it include increase in sexual libido, removal of wrinkles from the skin, relief from arthritic pain, prevention of ulcers, and cure of angina pectoris. From all the excitement, one would think that vitamin E was a new and wonderful discovery. The presence of vitamin E in food has been known for decades, but there has been no scientific evidence that it can fulfill any of these dramatic claims.

Vitamin E deficiency has been clinically observed only in very rare cases, in premature infants, who developed anemia and a skin irritation as a result.

Vitamin E is a chemical in the alcohol family and is soluble in fat. Its main function in the body is to work as a preservative, inhibiting the combination of a substance with oxygen. It is known to be essential in human beings, but a diet deficient in vitamin E produces no symptomatology of any disease. If you eat a normal, regular, fairly well-balanced diet, you will obtain all of the vitamin E that the body can use. It is found in abundant quantity in vegetable oils, margarine, wheat germ, leafy vegetables, and whole-grain cereals.

According to the Food and Drug Administration, any amount of vitamin E over 45 international units should be labeled as a drug. The daily requirement is considered to be 15 international units.

Vitamin K: Vitamin K is essential to the body's manufacture of a substance that helps to clot blood. Deficiency of vitamin K is rare, since it is found in abundance in a variety of foods, such as the green and leafy vegetables, tomatoes, eggs, soybean oil, and liver.

Perhaps the appropriate conclusion to the subject of vitamins is this clever poem given to me by one of the guests at La Costa:

> Vitamin A keeps the colds away
> and tends to make meek people nervy;
> B's what you need when you're going to seed,
> while C is specific for scurvy.

> Vitamin D makes the bones in your knee
> tough and hard for the service on Sunday;
> While E makes hens scratch and increases the hatch,
> and brings in more profits on Monday.

Vitamin F never bothered the Chef,
'cause that vitamin never existed;
G puts the fight in the old appetite,
and you eat all the foods that are listed.

So now when you dine, just remember these lines,
if long on this earth you would tarry.
Just try to be good and pick out more food
from the Garden, the Orchard, and Dairy.

It is important to remember that all of the essential nutrients — protein, carbohydrates, fats, vitamins, and minerals — are necessary to the proper functioning of your body, even when you are "dieting" to lose weight.

PART II

THE 14-DAY FOOD PLAN

Chapter 4

DIET AND WEIGHT CONTROL

The way people use the word *diet* has changed in recent years. The word actually means "daily sustenance," or a regular daily intake of food; but most people now think of it as what is left to them after all the really enjoyable foods have been taken away — a denial of food rather than a use of food.

Technically speaking, what I am presenting in this book is a "diet," but I do not want you to associate it with those foolish fad diets. What I am offering you is a guide to intelligent and sensible eating with which you can lose weight, gain weight, or maintain your weight. I want you to understand what food does to and for your body, so that you are in control of the way you look and the way you feel. For that reason I am going to call this a "food plan" rather than a diet. It may not sound as exciting as one of those fad diets that seem so easy and "fun" to follow because they oversimplify your food choices into one food grouping or another. But it is a much more *effective* plan, and when you come to understand what you are doing, it becomes much more enjoyable than following a fad could ever be, because *you* will be in control. You will be controlling your calories; they will not be controlling you.

Eat Anything You Want — in the Right Amount

Whether you want to gain weight, lose weight, or maintain your weight, the most important factor in your daily food regimen is keeping the proper balance of nutrients. You will probably be relieved to know that I do not intend to place any painful, worrisome, or severe restrictions on the foods you eat and enjoy. I do not want to deprive you of anything you like. I want you to be able to eat whatever foods you want, whenever you want — as long as you eat them in the right portions and proportions.

The only way you can be free to eat what you want is to know precisely what you are doing whenever you put a piece of food in your mouth. While eating is, and ought to be, a pleasurable experience, it is also nourishment for your body. What you should be doing when you eat is striking a balance between the joy of eating and the care and maintenance of the physical machine that is your body.

Comparing the human body to an automobile is an old analogy but a good one. Most of us wouldn't dream of mistreating our automobiles. They are expensive machines, and we are aware that the more we mistreat them the faster they will wear out and have to be replaced. So we are careful to give them the kind of fuel they need in the right amount, and we keep them supplied with oil, water, and everything else they need. Whenever there is the slightest thing wrong with them, we take them in to have the problem corrected.

Our bodies are far more important ''machines'' than our automobiles, yet we mistreat them much, much more. If our automobiles wear out, we can always replace them, even though it means some expense. If our bodies wear out, however, we cannot replace them no matter how much we are able to pay.

That analogy can be carried only so far; but it does hold true for the kind of damage that can be done to both machines by leaving them idle for too long, and it is very appropriate for the kind of damage caused by supplying each with the improper mixtures of fuels. Of course, a car does not get fat, but it may develop a cough and a sputter, and it may get its pipes and tubes clogged up.

No matter how intelligent or well educated you are, the most basic mechanical processes of your body may be a mystery to you. Most important, you are not aware of the proper way to eat. If you are an average American, you were probably given three rules to follow: sit up straight; keep your elbows off the table; and clean your plate. These are the wrong rules to follow, especially the last one, which has probably killed more Americans than all of the wars put together.

The truly important rules are: eat slowly; take small bites; masticate your food well (do not bolt your food and quickly wash it down with water — or worse, soda); and relax and enjoy your meal. These rules go hand in hand with what I have said about eating anything you want as long as it is the correct amount.

An interesting physiological fact is that the taste buds cease to function after the first few bites of any one food. After that, you are no longer satisfying the taste buds; instead, you have set up a texture pattern to the cortex of the brain that associates the texture of the food with the taste you enjoyed in the first few bites. What that means is that you do not have to eat a 16-ounce steak to get the pleasure out of eating a steak. You can eat much, much less and be just as satisfied — as long as you eat slowly and chew.

There are, of course, other reasons as well for eating slowly and chewing well. When you masticate your food, you start the enzymes functioning to help you digest the food properly. When you bolt your food, you are overloading the stomach and impairing the efficiency of the internal organs in breaking the food down into nutrients.

Unless you have some medical problem, you should be able to eat just about any kind of food you enjoy, as long as you remember that added piece of advice — the right *amount,* the right *portion,* the right *proportion.* Your body must have a balanced diet if it is to function well. The object of that balance is nutrition, getting the correct mixture of fuels so your body runs at top efficiency. Remember — a wide variety of foods in the proper amount.

What Is the Right Amount? (Your Calorie Level)

Many of us enjoy dining out in fine restaurants where the service is impeccable and the food is something to talk about. Generally, we are first ushered into the bar while waiting for our tables, and there we consume perhaps two martinis. Then we are escorted into a beautiful dining room with gorgeous linen and crystal; before we even get our menus, waiters bring hot loaves of bread accompanied by huge dishes of butter. We spread the bread generously with butter and munch on it while reading the menu. The food we order might be as follows: a crab cocktail, a bowl of soup, a salad with Roquefort dressing, a 16-ounce steak, a baked potato, and a small dish of vegetables. We might end the meal with a dish of chocolate ice cream.

This is what has become a "typical" American dinner in recent years. It contains approximately 3194 calories. Just to show you how severely you are overfueling your body when you eat such a meal, I will point out that that is the full day's caloric requirement for a 160-pound athlete or construction worker — and you are eating that amount in one meal!

An important part of the enjoyment of that meal is the variety of food and the slow, relaxed pace of dining. But the same pleasure and sense of luxury can be derived from smaller portions.

Many of the fad diets try to convince us that calories are not the problem with our excessive weight. No matter what claims they make and what gimmicks they use, calories are what they are working with in promising you weight loss.

Calories are a heat measurement; they are the way we measure the fuel that our body either utilizes as energy or stores as fat. We each need a specific number of calories each day in a specific balance of fat, carbohydrate, and protein. The exact number may vary from person to person, but the balance is virtually the same for all of us. Whatever the body takes in beyond our caloric level and out of balance — whether it is fat, carbohydrate, or protein — becomes stored in the body in the form of fat.

There is a popular misconception today — encouraged by irresponsible authors of fad diet books — that the way to lose weight is to emphasize one food group at the expense of the others. That is not true; the way to lose weight and to keep it off is to eat a balanced diet — balanced both in the percentages of the food groups and in the amount an individual needs for their specific life style.

The number of calories *you* need depends upon a number of individual factors — your age, sex, height, weight, and level of activity. If you came to my office at La Costa, I would have to take these factors into consideration in setting your level of calorie intake. Then, depending upon whether you wanted to lose or to gain weight, I would place you on a food plan. Since you are not in my office, you are going to have to make that determination for yourself, either alone or with the help of your doctor.

To set your calorie level, you will have to learn a few basic facts about your body and about how calories work.

HOW MUCH SHOULD YOU WEIGH?

There is some variation in what experts believe men and women of differing age groups and differing heights should weigh, and their recommendations have changed over the years, the standard weights generally becoming lower as people get less and less exercise. The most current and reliable figures appear in the table on page 33. The problem with such tables is that they are divided into categories of "small frame," "medium frame," and "large frame," and the individual should probably not be allowed to decide for himself or herself what kind of frame he or she has. Most likely, if you are overweight, you will try to make yourself feel better by assuming you have a large frame. It is best to let your doctor tell you what kind of frame you have and precisely what you should weigh.

However, if you are willing to be objective about yourself, you can estimate your bone structure by looking at your wrists and ankles. Since these are the parts of the body least likely to collect fat (and if you do by chance have fat wrists and ankles, you are so overweight it hardly matters to consider your frame), you can generally see just how big your bones really are. If you have small, delicate wrists, you have a small frame. If you have large wrists and ankles, you have a large frame. If you have difficulty in determining whether they are large or small, you are most likely in the "medium frame" category.

Even within the categories, you have a range of 10 to 15 pounds in which you can be considered reasonably fit. In the case of large frames, you have even more leeway. Fitness involves more than weighing the proper number of pounds for your height.

CHOOSING YOUR CALORIE LEVEL

The food plan I am presenting has three separate levels for you to choose from. You can lose weight from any of the three levels of calorie intake. Since I am also offering you an exercise program you can use for weight loss as well as for toning, it will be up to you (and perhaps your doctor) precisely how much weight you will lose, and how fast you will lose it.

From the table of desirable weights, you've already determined how overweight you are. Now decide exactly how much of that excess weight you want to lose immediately, say, in the first two weeks. How much in the following two weeks? How much of that do you think you can take care of with a brief daily program of exercise? How much do you want to lose strictly on the diet? Remember — losing weight should be steady and not too rapid, so that the body can compensate for the new weight.

The three levels of diet from which you can choose are 1200 calories, 1000 calories, and 800 calories. That is per day, not per meal. Don't worry, you won't go hungry. However, if you choose the 800-calorie-per-day diet, I prefer that you not stay on it for more than two weeks. After that time, you must go up to at least the 1000-calorie level because you will be losing some essential minerals at 800 calories. You should not stay on the 1000-calorie level for an extended period either. The 1200-calorie level will assure you of a widely varied and adequate intake of food.

At this point you have to use a bit of arithmetic, with or without a pocket calculator. Begin by getting on your scale and weighing yourself. The best time to do this is in the morning before breakfast. For an example, let us say your weight is 150 pounds. Next try to decide whether you are (1) very active, (2) active, (3) medium active, (4) mildly active, or (5) inactive. I know that is not easy to determine, so I will try to help you out: You are very active if you are an athlete or are involved in heavy physical labor for a large part of your day. You are active if you move about a great deal — for example, if you are a

HEIGHT — WEIGHT		
Height in inches	*Men*	*Women*
60	—	109 ± 9
62	—	115 ± 9
64	133 ± 11	122 ± 10
66	142 ± 12	129 ± 10
68	151 ± 14	136 ± 10
70	159 ± 14	144 ± 11
72	167 ± 15	152 ± 12
74	175 ± 15	—

(Heights and weights are without shoes and other clothing.)

Nutrition and Physical Fitness, *Bogert, Briggs, and Colloway. 1966, University of California.*

door-to-door salesperson or a letter carrier or a demonstrator of office equipment. You are medium active if you take care of children or work as a salesclerk in a store or teach school. You are mildly active if you work in an office and spend considerable time sitting at a desk. You are inactive if you do nothing all day, except perhaps move from your chair to the dining table and then to the television.

Now that you have decided your level of activity, you are going to do some multiplication. If you are very active, multiply your weight by 19; active, multiply by 17; medium active, multiply by 15; mildly active, multiply by 13; inactive, multiply by 11. Using our example of someone who weighs 150 pounds, let us say he or she falls into the medium active category. Multiplying by 15, we come up with 2250 calories — the amount of energy it takes for that person to get through each day without losing or gaining a pound. In short, you multiply your weight by your activity number to come up with the daily calorie consumption you need to maintain your present weight.

However, this figure is valid only if you are 25 years old or under. As we get older our metabolic requirements call for fewer calories, so we have to subtract calories for the metabolic slow-down. Age 25 is the peak metabolic year, and thereafter you require one percent fewer calories for each year over 25 to maintain your weight and bodily functions. This holds true until age 58. Above 58 we subtract one-third of the calorie requirements.

Let us compare, for example, the caloric requirements for a medium active person of 150 pounds at age 25 and at age 50:

25 years old	50 years old
150 lbs. optimum weight ×15 calories	150 lbs. optimum weight ×15 calories
2250 calories per day needed to maintain weight	2250.0 calories −562.5 calories (25%)
	1687.5 calories per day needed to maintain weight

Let us take another example of a medium active person whose optimum weight should be 200 pounds:

25 years old	50 years old
200 lbs. optimum weight ×15 calories	200 lbs. optimum weight ×15 calories
3000 calories per day needed to maintain weight	3000 −750 calories (25%)
	2250 calories per day needed to maintain weight

As I have pointed out, there are 3500 calories in each pound of stored fat. You must eat 500 calories less per day to lose one pound of weight per week, or 1000 calories less per day for a two-pound loss. A weight loss of two pounds per week sounds like a small amount but if continued would be more than 100 pounds per year. A greater weekly loss than this should be undertaken only with a physician's guidance.

In the previous example, the 25-year-old person consuming 2250 calories per day can lose one pound per week if he reduces his intake to 1750 calories per day, or 2 pounds per week if he eats 1250 calories per day.

The number of calories you cut out of your daily intake of food is known as your *calorie deficit*. If you want to know how much weight you will lose by cutting down your intake of food by, say, 500 calories per day, you multiply that number by the factor .002. Thus, 500 × .002 = 1 pound per week. If your calorie deficit is 1000 calories per day, then you will lose 1000 × .002 = 2 pounds per week. This method of predicting weight loss is found in the *Mayo Clinic Diet Manual* (pp. 71–73) and can be an aid in bringing to our attention how much we are overeating.

The calorie deficit is what makes you lose weight. If you have been overeating — consuming, say, 3000 calories per day — and are placed on a 1200-calorie diet, your calorie deficit is 1800 calories. 1800 × .002 = 3.6 pounds you could lose the first week. This is more than I consider safe but shows you that calorie deficit is important.

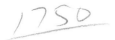

SALT AND SUGAR IN WEIGHT CONTROL

Salt, or sodium chloride, is one of the necessary nutrient minerals. Someone who weighs 150 pounds will have approximately 4 ounces of sodium in the body. It, together with potassium and chlorine, regulate what we refer to as the acid-alkali balance in the body.

However, the average American consumes between 10 and 20 grams of salt a day, about five times as much as do people in the rest of the world. The salt intake in this country is so extreme that most physicians consider it to be a definite health hazard. A large intake of salt is particularly harmful to people who have a history (or a family history) of high blood pressure (hypertension), because of the inherent danger of stroke or heart disease. It has been shown that low salt intake from childhood on can help to protect a person from hypertension.

Low salt intake is also very important in losing weight. Contrary to the popular myth, the body does not lose fat cells; that is physiologically impossible. The only way anyone can lose weight is to rid the fat cells of their contents and water (water comprises about 70 percent of the fat cell). To eliminate water from the fat cells, low sodium intake is essential.

To help reduce your intake of salt, I suggest:

1. Use herbs and spices to season your food in cooking, instead of using excessive salt.
2. Avoid heavily salted packaged foods such as potato chips, pretzels, nuts, and pickles.
3. Avoid processed foods that are high in salt as well as in sugar.
4. When a dish is served to you, do not salt it until you have tasted it to determine if it needs salt.

It is important to realize that you can get all the sodium you need naturally in the food you eat. It is not necessary to add salt to the food. If you feel salt is needed for taste, you can use a salt substitute — but read the label to make sure the substitute does not contain sugar.

I emphasized earlier that our bodies need two kinds of carbohydrates — starches and sugars. But by "sugar" I do not mean white table sugar (nor the kind of sugar found in molasses and honey). White table sugar is a nonfood; it supplies energy only. It has no vitamins and minerals, protein, or fat. Though it contains calories, they are considered "empty calories" that do not benefit the body. What the body *does* need are the starches and natural substances found in fruit and vegetables, milk and cereals, which the body will take and metabolize into the sugar it requires for energy.

The Senate Select Committee on Nutrition has issued a report recommending that the people of the United States reduce their salt consumption by 50 to 85 percent and their sugar consumption by 40 percent. (They further recommend that we reduce our fat consumption to less than 30 percent of our diet, while increasing our carbohydrate consumption up to 60 or 65 percent of the total.)

Our total sugar consumption *is* reaching staggering proportions. In 1910 the average person in the United States consumed approximately 73 pounds of sugar a year; but in 1971 that figure had risen to about 100 pounds of sugar per person per year.

If you feel you must have the sweet taste of sugar in your diet, use one of the sugar substitutes that is recommended by your physician.

As you grow to understand food and nutrition more fully, you should begin to see how you are "overnourishing" your body, whether it is with excessive salt, sugar, protein, or fat. With greater knowledge of food, you should be able to eat much more wisely.

While I will be setting forth a food plan for you (see Chapter 6), it will ultimately be up to you to control your eating habits. But before you get to the specific food plans you have to choose from, you need to acquaint yourself with the Exchange System, the method we use at La Costa for portion control.

Chapter 5

THE EXCHANGE SYSTEM

Most people find counting calories frustrating; they find it difficult to look at a dish of food in a restaurant and know how many calories it contains. But there is a simplified method of approximating calories. It is called the Exchange System, and it is based upon the internationally known diabetic exchange system designed to assist diabetics in selecting a well-balanced diet with a variety of foods. This system can be used with our slight modification by anybody who wants to control calories while still getting proper nutrition.

In this system, foods are divided into eight different lists or categories called "exchanges." You cannot substitute foods *between* these categories and maintain proper nutrition, but you can safely exchange any of the foods *within* each category in the amounts specified. In Chapter 6, where you will learn how to determine your food plan for weight loss, you will be breaking down your daily allowance of calories among the various exchanges, giving yourself one, two, or three meat exchanges at each meal, one or two vegetable exchanges, and so on. However, because it is so important that your body get the correct amount of calories in the proper balance of nutrients, you should eat precisely the exchanges specified in the amounts specified. Do *not* allow yourself to cheat by giving yourself a little extra meat, for example, at the expense of bread or vegetables, or you will be defeating the purpose of the plan. This system benefits anyone trying to lose weight because it assures you of getting all the essential nutrients. It is approved by all of the leading associations and research groups that are concerned with food and nutrition.

At first, it may seem just as difficult as any other system of calorie counting, but after the first few days of referring to tables you will begin to associate various foods automatically. If, for example, you know that you are permitting yourself one bread exchange, one vegetable exchange, two meat exchanges, one fruit exchange, and one skim milk exchange for a meal, you will find it easy to figure without having to turn to pencil and paper to total up calories.

In getting acquainted with the Exchange System, you may want to have some general understanding of how many calories of fat, carbohydrate, or protein each exchange represents. For that reason, the caloric values of each exchange are also indicated (in grams) for convenience and easy computation. One gram of carbohydrate or protein is always equal to 4 calories, and one gram of fat is always equal to 9 calories. You can now easily determine the calorie content of the foods you serve and eat.

For weighing foods, I suggest that you get a flat-top postal scale of good quality. There are 28.35 grams in an ounce, but I recommend rounding off the figure to 30 for your computations, since the difference is so insignificant.

Some of the lists of foods use various types of measurements; you may have to refer occasionally to the following list of standard measuring devices used in most household kitchens:

    3 teaspoons = 1 tablespoon
    8 tablespoons = ½ cup
    16 tablespoons = 1 cup = 8 fluid ounces
    16 ounces = 2 cups = 1 pint

    Iced tea glass = 12 ounces = 1½ cups
    Water goblet = 8 ounces = 1 cup
    Juice glass = 4 ounces = ½ cup

Measuring is important in this system. For example, a level teaspoon of sugar is 20 calories. A level teaspoon of milk is 11 calories. Skim milk has only 5 calories per teaspoon, while cream has 22 calories per teaspoon. If you use two teaspoons of cream (44 calories) plus one teaspoon of sugar (20 calories) in your coffee, each cup will cost you 64 calories. Multiply this by the number of cups of coffee you consume in a day, and you will find the number of calories are considerable. The nutrition in these calories is very low.

When you begin to plan your diet, when you shop and prepare your food, and when you have to dine out rather than at home, these exchange lists will come to have great meaning for you. While you are following your diet, at whatever caloric level, it is very important to remember these rules:

1. Eat only the amounts of the foods listed at your calorie level. More or less than these amounts will change the food value and calories proportionately.
2. Any additions (such as fats, starches, sauces, gravies, breadings, and sugars) to the foods as listed must be calculated for calorie content.
3. Eat regularly, slowly, in a quiet, pleasant atmosphere, with congenial companions. ''Stand-up'' eating is seldom satisfying.

These rules are important, simple, and easy to follow. The most important rule is the first: eat only the amounts permitted for your level. This is important because any alteration will affect the balance set up in the diet, and that balance is important for nutrition. To alter the amount of one food would mean juggling all of the foods on your menu. The second rule follows naturally from the first.

Rule 3 may not seem very important to you, but it is. Eating slowly gives your blood sugar time to rise, and it increases the satiety effect so that you can be much more satisfied with less food. Dining in a relaxing atmosphere and in pleasant company is also essential. Unfortunately, in America today, business and family problems are often discussed over a meal. Being overexcited while you are dining can cause you to eat more than you should and to poorly digest what you eat.

One evening I was explaining this to a group of guests at La Costa and a man in the back of the room said loudly, ''You mean I can't eat with my wife?'' He was joking, but there is a certain amount of truth in the joke. All too often the dinner table is the place where husband and wife share the troubles and worries they have had during the day. In a very short time, both are so upset that they cannot enjoy or digest their meal properly. Eating should be a pleasure, not a traumatic experience.

Vegetable Exchanges

Vegetables are divided into two lists of exchanges. All of those in the first list are what might be considered "watery" vegetables, and they are all exchanged at a measure of one cup, raw. Containing 3 grams of carbohydrate and 1 gram of protein, they total out at 16 calories for one cup. Although these vegetables do contain a small amount of protein, do not assume that all proteins are alike. Nutritionally, vegetable protein is not as valuable as animal protein, because vegetable protein is an incomplete protein.

The foods in this list average the same number of calories and the same food value if used in the same amount. These are the vegetables that you can use rather liberally. They are often used in salads, relish trays, vegetable soup, even in pot roast. They have considerable nutrient value, being high in both minerals and vitamins.

Don't let it disturb you if someone tells you that any of these vegetables — tomatoes, for example — are high in calories. This is not true, comparatively speaking, and it is the sort of distortion that can often be found in "popular" newsstand diet books.

List 1. Vegetable Exchanges

(1 cup raw measure)
3 grams carbohydrate + 1 gram protein = 16 calories

Asparagus
Bamboo shoots, bean sprouts
Beans: green string or
    yellow wax
Broccoli
Brussels sprouts
Cabbage
Cauliflower
Celery, celery leaves
Chinese cabbage
Cucumber
Eggplant
Greens: beet, chard, collard,
    dandelion, chicory, endive,
    kale, mustard,
    spinach, turnip

Kohlrabi
Mushrooms
Okra
Peppers: green, red, sweet, hot
Pimiento
Radish
Salad greens: lettuce, romaine,
    endive, curly endive,
    escarole, watercress
Sauerkraut
Green onion, scallion
Squash: zucchini, crookneck,
    summer squash
Tomato
Water chestnut

The List 2 vegetables, most of which are "root vegetables," are somewhat higher in caloric content than those in List 1. However, although they are higher, do not think you must stay away from them. They are the priceless vegetables that are very high in vitamins and minerals, so you must use them, but in the portion that fits your particular dietary need.

The List 2 vegetables are measured according to one-half cup cooked; and that measure contains 7 grams of carbohydrate and 2 grams of protein, giving a total of 36 calories. To realize how rich in calories they are, simply compare: one cup of the List 1 vegetables gives 16 calories; one-half cup of the List 2 vegetables gives 36. In other words, one-half the measure contains more than twice the calories.

List 2. Vegetable Exchanges

(½ cup cooked measure)
7 grams carbohydrate + 2 grams protein = 36 calories

> Artichoke (1 small, edible portion)
> Beets
> Carrots
> Leeks
> Onions
> Peas, green young tender
> Pumpkin
> Rutabaga
> Squash: winter, acorn, hubbard, butternut, banana
> Turnip

Fruit Exchanges

Fruits do not measure out the same as vegetables, so we have figured the amount of each fruit to equal 40 calories. Each portion represents 10 grams of carbohydrate, no extra sugar added. Our Spa dessert portions are also 40 calories, so if you do not like the desserts offered, you can easily substitute a fruit. Also, the 10-gram, 40-calorie portions of fruit seem to work out with a larger list of easily remembered portions — such as a whole small apple, a half a grapefruit, a whole orange, a peach, a pear, or two plums.

The carbohydrates in these fruits are often referred to as "fruit sugar." These sugars are much more nutritionally acceptable to the body than granulated table sugar, or glucose, from beets or sugar cane.

In shopping, remember that fruits and vegetables should be purchased when they are fully ripened, and at the height of the season, for this is when they are the most nutritious and delicious. Eye appeal plays a very important part in dieting, and, of course, in everyday living and eating. Choose, then, from among the fruit exchanges, an item that you really enjoy, that has eye appeal and is satisfying. Berries in season make an attractive dish, and you will notice that a 40-calorie serving of strawberries or blackberries is one cup. This amount fills about two-thirds of a cereal bowl. Dates and figs are higher in their percentage of sugar, so we get a smaller amount for 40 calories. This is applicable whether they are dried or fresh. Even though dried fruits weigh less, the calorie content is the same. The only thing that has been removed from the dried fruits is the water; the sugar remains.

Raisins are similarly misleading. On the golf course, I often see people carrying packages of raisins to have as a snack during the game. It is true that raisins are high in fruit sugar and are an excellent source of iron; but a handful of raisins can be eaten rather rapidly. Two level tablespoons of raisins are 40 calories. Because of their high caloric value, they should be measured carefully and used sparingly unless your dietary regime allows these additional calories.

In some cases, you may eat the entire fruit listed. The apple that you are permitted is what some people call a "schoolboy" apple — one small enough to fit easily into your pocket. A simple and easy way to measure such a fruit is to fit it into an average-size tea cup. In the case of bananas, which are relatively high in calories but which are also very nutritious, the amount that equals the allotted 40 calories is about one-half the average-size banana.

One of the popular diet books says that watermelon should never be used in a diet, and the author's reasoning is that no one ever stops with one piece. This is absurd, because the same statement could be made about almost every other type of food as well. Watermelon in the proper amount — a wedge about 4 by 1½ inches — is a very satisfying low-calorie dessert.

List 3. Fruit Exchanges

(No added sugar)
10 grams carbohydrates = 40 calories

Apple	1 small, 2½" diam.
Apple juice	⅓ cup
Applesauce	½ cup
Apricots, fresh	2 medium
cooked	½ cup
dried	4 halves
Banana	½ small (3")
Strawberries, blackberries	1 cup
Blueberries, boysenberries, gooseberries	⅔ cup
Loganberries, raspberries	½ cup
Cantaloupe	¼ of 6" melon
Cherries	10
Cranberry juice	1 cup (8 oz.)
Currants, fresh	⅔ cup
dried	1 tablespoon
Dates	2
Figs, fresh	1 large
dried	1 medium
Grapefruit	½ medium
Grapefruit juice	½ cup (4 oz.)
Grape juice	¼ cup
Grapes	12 medium to large
Guava	1 large or 3 small
Honeydew melon	⅛ of 7" melon
Kumquats	3 medium
Lemons	2 small or 1 large
Lemon juice	½ cup
Limes	2 medium or 3 small
Mango	¼

List 3. Fruit Exchanges (cont.)

Nectar, canned, apricot peach, pear	⅓ cup
Nectarine	1 medium
Orange, navel	1 medium
Valencia	1 small
Orange juice	½ cup, (4 oz.)
Papaya	⅓ medium
Peach	1 medium
Pear	1 medium
Persimmon	½ large
Pineapple, canned	½ cup chunks or 1 large slice
fresh	⅙ wedge of 4 × 6½-in. fruit
Plums	2 medium
Prune juice	¼ cup
Prunes, fresh or dried	2 medium
Raisins	2 Tbsp. level (1 oz.)
Rhubarb, cooked	1 cup
Tangerine	1 large
Watermelon	wedge, 4 × 1½-in. thick

Bread Exchanges

Here again, the portions have to vary somewhat. We have figured each of the bread exchanges to be equal to one slice of bread, or 68 calories. These 68 calories break down as 15 grams of carbohydrate and 2 grams of protein. Of course, each type of bread does have a slightly different value; but we do not want to complicate your diet beyond endurance, so we have generalized. (French bread, for example, is given a weight of 25 grams for an average piece of a presliced loaf from a bakery or supermarket.)

If you want to cut down your caloric value, buy a day-old unsliced loaf and slice it thinner than the average slice. At La Costa, we have done this with bagels, sometimes getting as many as twenty extremely thin slices out of one bagel. Toasted, they are excellent for nibbling. However, do not attempt to slice bagels at home. If you do want to try them, take your bagels to your butcher and ask him to slice them on his meat slicer.

It is not necessary to buy one of the many "diet" breads that are on the market. Diet breads do weigh less, some of them advertised as being 16 or 18 grams, because they are either raised higher or sliced thinner. Bite for bite and weight for weight, diet breads have approximately the same food value as regular bread, so you need not to restrict yourself to them. We want you to have as much freedom and flexibility in your diet as possible.

In the bread exchange, we include cereals, biscuits, rolls, corn bread, flour, and potatoes. Since flour is necessary in thickening various types of sauces, you need to know the number of calories in the thickener.

The average cooked cereal is about 68 calories for a half-cup, but the dry packaged cereals vary so widely in calories that you must shop very carefully. Almost all of the dry cereals today have added sugar, and many of them also have added salt. With the new nutritional labeling (see page 74) required by the Food and Drug Administration, any additions to or subtractions from a packaged food must be identified on the label.

Sugar added to a dry cereal often doubles the caloric value of the product. It has also become popular to add numerous vitamins and minerals to breakfast cereals, and these additions raise the price of the cereal. When you eat your breakfast cereal, you may in effect be taking a vitamin supplement that you don't really need — and paying for it, too.

Nutrition Action, a publication of the Center for Science in the Public Interest, reports in the July 1975 issue on the concern of health professionals about a new cereal that contains 110 calories, with only one gram of protein and a sugar content of 40 to 50 percent. In order to circumvent the law about nutritional labeling, the article explains, the manufacturers group the four flours in the product as "cereal grain." They then list the three sweeteners separately as sugar, brown sugar, and corn syrup. The result is that a quick glance at the label will make the consumer think he is getting more nutrition than he actually is.

A few vegetables are included in the bread exchanges; note carefully that a white potato has half the caloric value of a sweet potato, and note also that you can have a fairly good sized piece of angel food cake for 68 calories. If you are having a birthday party, the candles will burn just as brightly on an angel food cake as they will on a German chocolate cake at 400 calories per slice.

List 4. Bread Exchanges

---

15 grams carbohydrate + 2 grams protein = 68 calories

Bread, white, French, Italian, wheat, rye, pumpernickel	1 slice (25 grams)
Bagel	½ medium (3″ diameter)
Biscuit or roll	1 (2″ diameter)
Bread crumbs, dry, grated	¼ cup
soft	⅓ cup
Bread sticks	2 (6½″ long)
Buns, frankfurter or hamburger	½
Cake, angel food	1 slice (1½″ at edge)
Cereal, cooked	½ cup
Cereal, dry packaged	(Wide variation in calories from 55 to 200 per serving. Read label.)
Rice or grits, cooked	½ cup
Corn bread	1½″ cube
Crackers	
Graham	2
Oyster	½ cup
Holland Rusk	2
Saltines	5
Soda	3
Thin, small	6 to 8
Zwieback	2½
Flour	2½ Tbsp. level
Barley	1½ Tbsp.

List 4. Bread Exchanges (cont.)

Cornstarch	2 Tbsp. level
Tapioca, dry	2 Tbsp.
Macaroni, noodles, spaghetti, cooked	½ cup
Matzo.	1 (5″ square)
Matzo meal	3 Tbsp.
Muffin, English	½ (3″ diam.)
Muffin, plain	1 small (2″ diam.)
Toast, Melba	4 rectangles or 8 rounds
Tortilla, corn	1 (6″ diameter)
Beans, dried, cooked	½ cup
Corn, ear	½ large or 1 small
Corn, whole kernel	⅓ cup
Parsnip	1 medium
Peas, dried, cooked	½ cup
Potato, white	1 small (2″ diameter)
Potato, sweet, or yam	½ of 1 small (2″ diameter)

Meat Exchanges

This is the first exchange to include fat, and it includes only meats that have no fats added to them in processing. The caloric value of fat is 2¼ times that of carbohydrates or proteins. (Remember, there are 9 calories per gram of fat as compared with 4 calories per gram of protein or carbohydrate.) These are the concentrated foods, and the portions used must be planned carefully so that they will be adequate and yet not exceed your caloric requirements.

One meat exchange (one ounce) is 73 calories and contains 7 grams (28 calories) of protein and 5 grams (45 calories) of fat. This might seem to you to be a fairly fatty piece of meat, but it is not; it is one ounce of lean trimmed meat. Everything on this exchange is calculated to exchange for one ounce of meat. Poultry, liver, and fresh fish (other than shellfish) are all averaged at 73 calories an ounce, cooked weight. (Meat shrinks by approximately one-third its weight when cooked because of loss of water.)

On a restaurant menu, the weight listed is raw weight, trimmed and ready for the cook. A 10-ounce filet steak, then, would be approximately 7 ounces when served, and it would have a caloric value of approximately 511 calories. This would be about seven meat exchanges. However, in many restaurants, before a steak is served, the cook melts one or two pats of butter on it to make it look shiny and appetizing, thereby raising its caloric value by 45 to 90 calories.

Some cold cuts are processed, and they vary widely in the addition of fats, spices, soybean extenders, cereals, and such. Most of them are precooked, and we average them here as one slice being 4½ inches square by ⅛ inch thick. One frankfurter of the all-meat variety is considered to be one meat exchange. Codfish, salmon, tuna, and swordfish are all fatty fish, and one piece approximately 2 by 2 inches exchanges for one ounce of cooked meat.

Shellfish contain much less fat, so with oysters, shrimp, or clams you may have five small or three large (or approximately 1½ ounces) to exchange for one ounce of meat.

The meat exchanges include other foods that are high in protein and contain fat — foods such as cheese, eggs, and peanut butter — and that are all quite nutritional. The various cheeses vary in fat content and moisture content as well as in their aging processes, so the equivalent relationship can only be approximated. For convenience, the values of the seventeen most popular varieties of cheese have been averaged at 73 calories per ounce. Most cheese packages have the accurate weight on the package. The precut foil-wrapped triangles usually come in one-ounce sizes. Cream cheese is included not in the meat exchanges but in the fat exchanges.

The cheeses we include here are excellent sources of protein, minerals, and fat-soluble vitamins. Since much of the water content of cheese is drained off in the whey, cheese is a concentrated food that compares quite favorably with meat in nutrient value. (It takes 10 pounds of milk to produce one pound of American cheese.) However, cheese is low in iron.

Creamed cottage cheese is a soft, unaged cheese; it is moistened either with whole milk (3.6 percent fat) or low-fat milk (2 percent fat). Dry cottage cheese is moistened with skim milk. Cottage cheese is an excellent food, but it is not low in calories. It is used extensively in diets in which the protein content must be high and the fat content low.

One large Grade A egg exchanges for one ounce of meat. The yolk of an egg contains 51 calories and most of the fat, minerals, and vitamins. The egg white is pure albumen and contains 22 calories. It is best to eat eggs that are cooked because the raw egg white contains an element which destroys vitamins.

Peanut butter is nutritious food, but it is high in calories. There are approximately 600 calories in 100 grams (3⅓ ounces). The percentage of protein, fat, and carbohydrate in peanut butter compares favorably with the meats and the cheeses. It contains considerable calcium, phosphorus, iron, sodium, and potassium.

When I was a young boy, peanut butter was simply crushed peanuts. As the merchandisers of peanut butter became more astute, they homogenized it to make it smooth, and then they hydrogenated it to make it soft, so that you could apply more to your bread or crackers.

Young people today have reverted back to the uncomplicated ''natural'' foods, so every manufacturer of peanut butter now makes an ''old-fashioned'' peanut butter along with its standard modern brands. If you buy a pound of the old-fashioned peanut butter and allow it to sit on a shelf for a while, you can then pour off a considerable amount of oil (part of the fat content), thereby reducing the caloric value and allowing you to have almost twice as much peanut butter without sacrificing the protein content.

List 5. Meat Exchanges.

(Lean, no fat added)
7 grams protein + 5 grams fat = 73 calories

Meat, poultry, liver, fresh fish, no bone	1 slice, lean
Cooked weight, 1 oz.; raw weight, 1⅓ oz.	
Cold cuts	1 slice (1½" sq. or diameter × ⅛")

List 5. Meat Exchanges (Cont.)

Canadian bacon	2 thin slices (1 oz.)
Cheese, cheddar, Swiss, American .	1-oz. slice (3½ × 3½ × ⅛ in.)
Creamed cottage cheese	¼ cup
Low-fat cottage cheese	½ cup
Parmesan, grated	3 Tbsp. level
Egg	1 large
Anchovies, no oil	9 thin fillets
Anchovy paste	2 Tbsp. level
Caviar, no oil	2 Tbsp. level (1 oz.)
Clams, oysters, shrimp	5 small or 3 large
Crab, lobster	⅓ cup (1½ oz.)
Herring, pickled	1 piece 1 × 1½ × 1½ in.
Lox, no oil	1 oz.
Sardines, no oil	3 medium
Scallops	2–3 (1½ oz.)
Frankfurter	1 (8 to 10 per lb.)
Peanut butter	2 Tbsp. level

Fat Exchanges

All of the foods listed in the fat exchanges are figured to be the equivalent of one pat (one level teaspoon) of butter, which is 5 grams of pure fat. Each of these foods supplies 45 calories, a surprisingly large number of calories for one tiny pat, but remember that pure fat is a highly concentrated food.

Because of this high concentration, fats should be used with discretion and they should be accurately measured. A butter cutter is a valuable tool; it will cut a quarter-pound of butter into twelve pats, so that you will know precisely how much you are getting, with no guesswork involved.

Certain fats and oils are essential to a balanced diet. The fats in the meat exchanges will give you all that you need of saturated fat. However, you also require some polyunsaturated fatty acid, one of which — linoleic acid — is extremely important to the body in small amounts. Linoleic acid cannot be synthesized or manufactured by the body, so it must be taken in through food.

Saturated fats are often called "hard fats" and are of animal origin; butter, meat, eggs, and, of course, hard margarine. Polyunsaturated fatty acids come from vegetables and are found in such sources as corn oil, peanut oil, and vegetable-oil margarine. A diet high in saturated fats is often associated with a high blood cholesterol.

Most of the unsaturated fats are liquid at room temperature (the most notable exception is coconut oil, which is liquid but highly saturated). The manufacturers of the hard cooking fats and margarines depend upon the addition of hydrogen to make their products hard. Hydrogen destroys their value as a source of linoleic acid. In cooking, use liquid vegetable oils or those labeled polyunsaturated. A polyunsaturated margarine should list "pure" liquid safflower, corn, soybean, or cottonseed oil as the first or predominant ingredient. Soft margarines have been whipped with an addition of air and water. Being soft, they are likely to be used in large quantities by the consumer. Read the label carefully, because this is the only way you can be certain whether or not the product meets your requirements. The calorie count per teaspoon, the kind of oil, and all of the other ingredients should be listed clearly on the label.

The total fat content of the average American diet may be as much as 41 to 50 percent of the total calories consumed per day. I feel this amount should be reduced to approximately 30 percent of your total calories. You should also substitute polyunsaturated oils and fats for part of your saturated fats. One to three ounces of polyunsaturated fat a day will meet the requirements of an adequate diet.

You may be surprised to see that bacon, coconut, cream cheese, salad dressings, mayonnaise, nuts, olives, and avocados are listed in the fat exchanges. Side bacon furnishes very little except fat, so if you enjoy the flavor of smoked meats, choose lean ham or lean Canadian bacon; they will offer you more protein. Cream cheese does not have the protein content that is furnished by the other cheeses, so it must be considered a fat exchange rather than a meat exchange. It is usually used for a spread as a substitute for butter or margarine or jelly. Neufchâtel is a low-fat cream cheese, and it is quite acceptable as a substitute, having half the caloric value of the full cream cheeses. Processed cheeses, which include the cheese spreads, are made from water, whey, dry milk solids, artificial color, and preservatives. There is wide variation in the caloric value and sodium and fat content of these cheeses, so you should read the labels.

Various types of cream vary in fat content and caloric value according to the amount of milk they contain. Restaurants usually serve half-and-half for use in coffee and cereal. Half-and-half contains about 11 percent butterfat, with the remainder being fluid milk. You should avoid this cream in your coffee because of the fat content. For coffee, skim milk is seldom satisfactory to most people, but whole milk can certainly be used. The vegetable-oil products that are used as nondairy coffee creamers are just as high in calories as the cream they substitute for. One teaspoon of powdered creamer is equal to one tablespoon of 20 percent cream (22 calories). Some of these creamers are made of coconut oil, which is as highly saturated as butter.

Formerly, "coffee cream" was 20 percent cream, and whipping cream was 40 percent cream. Now, because of increased prices and because of the general concern about high fat in diets, you can rarely find 40 percent cream; instead, 20 percent cream is sold as an all-purpose cream. With the advent of the aerosol can, it became possible to have whipped cream with a lower fat content. Sour cream, which is used in a great many salad dressings, is a cultured product with about 20 percent butterfat.

Salad dressings are fat exchanges, and they can be divided into two categories. The thin salad dressings are variations of oil and vinegar, or oil with lemon juice and condiments. The thick dressings are those made either with sour cream or with a mayonnaise base. The thick dressings are much higher in calories, so the thin dressings are preferable. Another advantage of the thin dressings is that when salads are mixed in a large serving bowl with the dressing, much of the dressing is left in the serving bowl when the salad is served into the smaller dishes.

An average serving of thin dressing has only one or two teaspoons of oil, making it somewhere between 45 and 90 calories. The average restaurant serving of thick dressing is one-fourth of a cup, which is about 12 teaspoons. Multiplying those 12 teaspoons by 45 (the number of calories in a level teaspoon of mayonnaise), we arrive at the astounding figure of 640 calories of fat for each serving of a thick Thousand Island or Roquefort dressing.

Nuts are listed in the fat exchanges, and they are very valuable as a source of polyunsaturated fat. However, shelled nuts tend to be consumed at a rather rapid and careless rate. A handful of shelled peanuts can easily be as many as forty to fifty nuts, and that can add up to a great many calories. I recommend that you buy nuts in the shell. They average about 7 calories each (six small nuts being about 45 calories). Since it takes time to crack the shells and eat the nuts, the taste of nuts is in your mouth for just as long a time as it would be if you had eaten one handful after another of shelled nuts. When serving nuts in the shell, if you accompany them with a bulky fruit such as grapes, apples, pears, or dried fruits, you can have a very nutritious and satisfying dessert for somewhere between 85 and 100 calories.

The shelled nuts that are labeled "dry roasted" are equal in calories to nuts in the shell. The regular salted nuts are likely to be roasted in oil, and, of course, the caloric value rises proportionately.

Olives are an oily fruit, usually cured by soaking in an alkali and then rinsing and curing in a salt brine. Very little oil is lost in curing, and each olive contains between 10 and 15 calories, depending on size.

Although avocados are very high in vegetable fat, a half an avocado about 4 inches in diameter (making it about 180 calories) can be used as a main course when filled with crab meat, lobster, or fruit (bringing it to 250 calories). If you fill it with low-fat cottage cheese and garnish with fresh pineapple wedges, again you will have a fairly well balanced meal at around 350 calories

List 6. Fat Exchanges

5 grams fat = 45 calories

Butter or margarine	1 pat (1 tsp. level)
Bacon, crisp	1 slice
Coconut, fresh	1 piece 1 × 1 × ⅜ in.
Cream Cheese	1 Tbsp. level
Neufchâtel cheese	2 Tbsp. level
Cream, light (20%)	2 Tbsp. level
heavy (40%)	1 Tbsp. level
French dressing or oil and vinegar .	1 Tbsp.
Mayonnaise	1 tsp. level
Nuts in shell	6 small
Tartar sauce	2 tsp. level
Oil or cooking fat	1 tsp.
Olives	5 small or 3 large
Avocado	⅛ (4″ diameter)

Milk Exchanges

The carbohydrate contribution to an 8-ounce glass of whole milk is halfway between a fruit exchange and a bread exchange. The protein in an 8-ounce glass of milk exchanges for an ounce of meat, a half cup of low-fat cottage cheese, or an egg. The fat is about 10 grams, or the equivalent of two pats of butter. The number of calories in a glass of milk is 170 (containing 12 grams of carbohydrate, 8 grams of protein, and 10 grams of fat).

Milk is considered by some to be a perfect food, and it does have a tremendous amount of nutritional value. It is especially valuable as a source of calcium and fat-soluble vitamin A. The protein found in milk is a complete protein, and most of the essential amino acids are present in the percentage needed by humans. Milk also contains minerals that are necessary for life, such as phosphorus, potassium, and sodium.

One of the major shortcomings of milk as a ''perfect food'' is that it contains practically no iron and very little vitamin C, and is also low in niacin and vitamin B_{12}. The vitamin D added to milk is negligible. Because of the lack of iron and vitamin C, an infant who is not breast-fed must have its diet fortified early with these two nutrients. An infant's iron stores at birth will probably last the first four months of life, by which time orange juice and whole-grain or fortified cereal can be added to its diet.

List 7. Whole Milk Exchanges

12 grams carbohydrate + 8 grams protein + 10 grams fat = 170 calories

Milk, whole	1 cup (8 oz.)
Milk, evaporated	½ cup
Powdered whole milk, dry	⅓ cup
Yogurt (whole milk)	1 cup (8 oz.)

Skim milk, or nonfat milk, contains only 0.1 percent fat, while retaining the same amount of carbohydrate (12 grams) and protein (8 grams) as whole milk. With the fat removed, the caloric value is less than half that of whole milk, 80 calories. All of the nutrients remain in skim milk, except for the fat-soluble vitamins A and D. These are generally replaced in the processing, and the product is then called ''fortified'' skim milk.

The American Heart Association has recommended for years that adults completely remove from their diets whole milk and cheeses made from whole milk and cream, and substitute skim milk and the cheeses made from skim milk. They point to the epidemic of coronary heart disease, and to studies which reveal that saturated fat, cholesterol, and high-calorie diets contribute to atherasclerosis and heart disease.

Remember when you pick up a glass of whole milk that you are getting not only all of the vitamins, minerals, and nutritional benefits of skim milk, but also the equivalent of two pats of butter. At first you may not find skim milk as ''rich-tasting'' as whole milk, but if you stay on it for a few weeks, you probably cannot go back to whole milk. Reducing the risk of contributing to heart disease is well worth the switch.

List 8. Skim Milk Exchanges

12 grams carbohydrate + 8 grams protein = 80 calories

Skim milk, nonfat (0.1% fat)	1 cup
Buttermilk, made from skim	1 cup
Dry cottage cheese	¾ cup
Powdered skim milk, dry	⅓ cup

The foods in this list are not a part of the exchange system. They are included here only because people are always asking about them. Sugar, of course, is a major concern to most people. Notice that one teaspoon of sugar is 20 calories, exactly the same number as honey. Honey is no more a "health" food than is plain sugar, and it is no easier to digest than plain sugar.

Ice creams are difficult to discuss because they are controlled by individual states, so I have to generalize here. However, a quarter of a pint of ice cream can usually be figured as approximately equal to one-half cup and 158 calories. Sherbet is somewhat lower, but not as low as many people think; it averages about 130 calories per half cup. Many of the dietetic ice creams are sweetened with sorbitol, which is a sweetener that is slower to metabolize than sugar.

Sweetened gelatin, as you can see, is relatively high in calories — 78 calories for one-half cup. The American public has long been led to believe that gelatin desserts, as well as cottage cheese, is exceedingly low in calories. They are both quite high in calories; but while cottage cheese is nutritional and an excellent meat substitute, gelatin desserts have very few useful calories. They are usually little more than sugar water, and the average restaurant adds a generous topping of whipped cream, making the gelatin dessert as high in calories as a small piece of apple pie.

However, you can buy small packages of plain, unsweetened gelatin that can be used in making low-calorie desserts with one, two, or three fruit exchanges (see the dessert recipes in chapter 16).

Miscellaneous Foods

List 9. Miscellaneous Foods

Sugar	1 tsp. level = 20 calories
Honey	1 tsp. level = 20 calories
Ice cream (¼ pint)	½ cup = 158 calories
Sherbet (¼ pint)	½ cup = 130 calories
Sweetened gelatin dessert	½ cup = 78 calories
Dietetic ice cream (sweetened with sorbitol only, ¼ pint)	½ cup = 85 calories

Foods Allowed as Desired

Many diets have what they call "free" foods — those you can have as much of as you want whenever you want. Nutritionally, there is no such thing, because all nutritional foods have calories that your body must use in some way or turn into fat. You can, however, have seasonings, certain condiments, and spices without having to calculate how they will affect your energy and calorie levels. The following are those you can use "freely":

Artificial noncalorie sweeteners	Spices
Plain coffee or tea	Rennet tablets
Unsweetened gelatin	Vanilla
Seasonings	Vinegar

Chapter 6

THE PLANS FOR WEIGHT LOSS

In setting about your sensible and well-ordered balanced diet, you will be given a wide variety of foods to choose from. On pages 145 through 158, you will find menus for luncheon and dinner for fourteen days. Each menu offers you a selection of appetizers, salads, entrées, vegetables, and desserts. The recipes for preparing each of these dishes can be found in Chapter 16, at the end of the book. All of these recipes and menus will apply to you whether you are on the 800-, the 1000-, or the 1200- calorie diet; it is simply the amount of each dish that may vary.

After fourteen days, you may repeat the menus, or you may be able to work up your own menus using the dishes and recipes offered. Even after you return to "normal" living, you may enjoy eating these dishes to maintain weight. Guests, too, will enjoy them. More generous portions may be served to guests with other items such as bread, butter, milk, and such.

Except for breakfast, for which you will have a single menu to use for the entire fourteen days, you will have menus that are separated into soups and appetizers, salads, entrées, vegetables, and desserts. The menus show the number of calories per serving of each dish. You will, of course, have to tally up the total number of calories of your selections to see that they match your calorie allowance for the meal.

For example, let us say you are on the 800-calorie diet. On the first dinner menu, should you select Vegetable Soup to begin (50 calories), follow that with the Italian Salad Bowl (25 calories), then Medallion of Veal Princesse (146 calories) and Ratatouille (16), finishing up with the Coupe St. Jacques (40 calories), your total number of calories is 277. On the 800-calorie diet, you are allowed 276 calories for dinner; you are only one calorie over your allowance, so you are all right. However, should you have chosen the Fresh Artichoke with Hot Dip (36 calories) rather than the Ratatouille, you would have been 21 calories over your limit, and that is a significant number, not to be dismissed lightly. (If you think 21 extra calories is insignificant, multiply that by 365 days a year. The total extra for a year would be 7,665 calories — more than two pounds of fat you do not need.)

On the same menus, you are instructed to select from "appetizers," "salads," "entrées," and so on, just as from a regular menu. However, as you consider your meals in the normal way, I am going to ask you to consider your calories in such a way that you will begin to get acquainted with what you are eating. Not only will you be totaling up your calories for each meal, you will also be considering "food exchanges."

The Exchange System, which was explained in Chapter 5, is a method of approximating calories as you balance your foods among fats, carbohydrates, and proteins. In selecting from your menus, you will be exchanging foods according to this system. In doing this, whether you realize it or not, you will be counting calories and balancing your menus.

If left to his own devices, the average American will choose a meal that is 20 percent protein, 40 percent carbohydrate, and 40 percent fat. This meal is far too high in fat content, no matter what your calorie level is. The balance of percentages does change depending upon the calorie level you require, largely because of the amount of protein a body needs. No one should have less than 50 grams of protein in a day, nor should anyone go above 65 grams of protein a day. (Although some highly active adults can use up to 70 grams of protein per day). Above that amount, the excess is automatically turned into fat.

The term *high protein* can be misleading. Meals that are high in protein can be very good for you — within limits. As long as your total calorie intake is below 2500 calories, your percentage of proteins should be relatively high. In higher-calorie diets, however, the percentages of protein and fat become less, and the carbohydrate percentage increases.

The confusion, for most people, occurs in the assumption that meat is pure protein. Lean meat is only about 26 percent protein and about 17 percent fat, and the remainder is taken up by water, gristle, vessels, and nonnutritive tissue. There are only 7 grams of protein in one ounce of meat. If you consume 10 ounces of meat a day, you are getting 70 grams of protein, most likely more than your body needs for building. If you are getting that amount at the expense of your carbohydrate intake, you are straining your body by making it convert the extra protein to carbohydrate (by the process known as gluconeogenesis).

Also, you should remember that you do not get all of your protein from meat. Some comes from cheese, eggs, milk, and bread and vegetables.

Interestingly, a good balance for reasonable calorie intake is found in milk. Although there is no such thing as a "complete" food, milk is the closest thing we have to one. The balance of the three food groups in whole milk is: 27 percent protein, 40 percent carbohydrate, and 33 percent fat. This is not a bad balance for the total amount of calories used by an infant. But I feel that a reasonable, safe, and sane diet for an adult should attempt to keep the protein below 25 percent and the fat below 30 percent, with the remainder taken up by carbohydrates. (The breakdown of fat should be about one-third saturated and two-thirds polyunsaturated.)

Americans have long depended upon meat as the main staple of diet, so it is now difficult for most people to keep the protein and fat content of their meals to the levels I recommend. However, for the sake of survival, I feel we must all try to do this.

The calorie levels I recommend for weight loss do vary slightly from the ideal percentages of proteins, carbohydrates, and fats, principally because adjustments have been made to see that you also get the essential vitamins and minerals. It is impossible to get all of the necessary nutrients into your diet each day on less than 1200 calories. You can, however, manage without fats until your own stored fat has been used and without some of the vitamins and minerals for a *limited* period of time, so long as you do make up that deficiency soon after a strict diet.

The 800-Calorie Level

At 800 calories, you will be eating just about everything you normally eat — only less of it. You will have bread, meat, fruit, vegetables, milk, and even eggs if you want them. However, do not think you can leave out one thing on the diet and then double up on something else. That is cheating and it is not allowed. The object is variety, to get all of the proper nutrition and the full benefit of a balanced diet. You will have choices within each of the exchanges, but you must eat three meals a day in the proportions laid out.

Your daily calorie breakdown is 264 calories for breakfast, 260 calories for lunch, and 276 calories for dinner.

Breakfast: The breakfast is the same for all three diet levels, and you are permitted a very wide choice of food. (See the menu on page 144.)

According to the Exchange System (see Chapter 5), you are permitted:

(A) One bread exchange,
(B) One meat exchange,
(C) One fruit exchange, and
(D) One skim milk exchange.

Selecting your breakfast from the menus, this breaks down roughly into a fairly standard breakfast. For example, you can choose the following way:

(A) Fruit or juice,
(B) Two eggs *or* a steak *or* one egg and cottage cheese, and
(C) One slice of toast with diet jam or jelly.

Or you can combine your selection to have:

(A) Fruit or juice,
(B) Cereal with nonfat milk,
(C) Cottage cheese *or* an egg, and
(D) One slice of toast with diet jam or jelly.

You can, of course, have coffee or tea with your breakfast, but you should not add sugar or cream. Use a sugar substitute if you wish, and take some milk from your milk allowance.

If you study the exchange tables, you will see that you are getting carbohydrate from your fruit exchange and your bread exchange; you are getting protein from your bread exchange, your meat exchange, and your skim milk exchange; and you are getting fat from your meat exchange. The balance is fairly good, even though your total calories are fairly low.

Lunch: Your 260-calorie lunch gives you:

(A) Two List 1 vegetable exchanges,
(B) Two meat exchanges,
(C) One List 2 vegetable exchange, and
(D) One fruit exchange.

On the menu, this translates roughly into one appetizer, one salad, one entrée, one vegetable, and one dessert. For this meal, at 800 calories, you do not get a bread exchange or a milk exchange. Look over the luncheon menus (beginning on page 145), and you will see that each menu entry is accompanied by a calorie count. Since the menus are prepared for all three calorie levels, you

THE 800-CALORIE LEVEL

Meal	Carbohydrate (46%)	Protein (26%)	Fat (28%)
Breakfast:			
Milk	12 gms = 48 cals	8gms = 32 cals	———
Meat	———	7 gms = 28 cals	5 gms = 45 cals
Bread	15 gms = 60 cals	2 gms = 8 cals	———
Fruit	10 gms = 40 cals	———	———
	37 gms = 148 cals	17 gms = 68 cals	5 gms = 45 cals
Luncheon:			
List 1 Veg.	6 gms = 24 cals	2 gms = 8 cals	———
List 2 Veg.	7 gms = 28 cals	2 gms = 8 cals	———
Meat	———	14 gms = 56 cals	10 gms = 90 cals
Fruit	10 gms = 40 cals	———	———
	23 gms = 92 cals	18 gms = 72 cals	10 gms = 90 cals
Dinner:			
List 1 Veg.	3 gms = 12 cals	1 gm = 4 cals	———
List 2 Veg.	7 gms = 28 cals	2 gms = 8 cals	———
Meat	———	14 gms = 56 cals	10 gms = 90 cals
Fruit	20 gms = 80 cals	———	———
	30 gms = 120 cals	17 gms = 68 cals	10 gms = 90 cals
Total	90 gms = 360 cals	52 gms = 208 cals	25 gms = 225 cals

(*Total Calories:* 793)

will have to total up various combinations to see that your combination will give you the correct number of calories.

Most of the entrées, both at lunch and dinner, total 146 calories, precisely two meat exchanges. Occasionally there will be an entrée that is higher, such as Linquini with Clam Sauce or Tostada. However, these include some bread and vegetable exchanges as well as meat. What you do is cut down on bread and vegetable to have the higher-calorie entrée. Total up the various combinations of courses to get what you want as close to 260 calories as possible. Learning is part of the fun of this diet.

Dinner: You get your largest meal at dinner — 276 calories. In terms of exchanges, the dinner breaks down as follows:

    (A) Two fruit exchanges,
    (B) Two meat exchanges,
    (C) One List 1 vegetable exchange, and
    (D) One List 2 vegetable exchange.

On the menus, you get your choice of one appetizer, one salad, one entrée, one vegetable, and one dessert. In your lunch and dinner, you are getting carbohydrate in both your List 1 and your List 2 vegetables, and in your fruit;

you are getting protein in both of the vegetables and in the meat; and you are getting fat in the meat. All three food groups in a fairly good balance.

Snacks: You are not allowed between-meal snacks at 800 calories. However, if you are terrified that you may starve to death in the middle of the night, take a piece of fruit to bed with you. Just remember, however, that that piece of fruit represents 40 calories, so you are not to take a bite out of it unless you have to reach out with your last dying gasp to get it to stay alive!

I recall one guest at La Costa who protested so vigorously against the 800-calorie level I had placed her on that I permitted her to take an apple with her to her room each night. At the end of her two-week stay, she was so pleased with her ability to restrain herself from eating them that she proudly presented me with fourteen rather sad-looking apples. She had found she hadn't needed them, but it had comforted her to know that they were there.

It may benefit you to see where you are getting your nourishment, and how the balance of food groups comes out. Of course, we cannot be precise, because the Exchange System is a method of approximating calories. But a glance at the table on page 55 will show you just about where you are getting your breakdown of proteins, carbohydrates, and fats. While your various exchanges are often mixed into salads, appetizers, and entr´ees on most menus, it will benefit you to see in exact figures that meat is not pure protein — that a very large percentage of even the leanest meat is fat.

The 1000-Calorie Level

The major difference between the 800-calorie level and the 1000-calorie level is that you get more of a bread exchange and milk exchange in your daily allowance, and you get more leeway in selecting your entrées. The calorie breakdown for the day is 264 calories for breakfast, 362 calories for lunch, and 346 calories for dinner.

Breakfast: At 1000 calories, the breakfast remains the same as at 800 calories — 264 calories. (See page 144.)

Luncheon: With lunch, you get 362 calories, divided loosely into:

(A) One bread exchange,
(B) Two meat exchanges,
(C) Two List 1 vegetable exchanges,
(D) One List 2 vegetable exchange, and
(E) Two fruit exchanges.

In selecting from the luncheon menu, give yourself:

(A) One appetizer,
(B) One salad,
(C) One entrée,
(D) One bread exchange,
(E) One vegetable, and
(F) One dessert.

You can select your bread exchange from List 4 on page 43, remembering that it is the equivalent of one slice of bread.

Dinner: On the 1000-calorie level, your dinner rises to 346 calories.

The 1000-CALORIE LEVEL

Meal	Carbohydrate (56%)	Protein (22%)	Fat (22%)
Breakfast:			
Milk	12 gms = 48 cals	8 gms = 32 cals	———
Meat	———	7 gms = 28 cals	5 gms = 45 cals
Bread	15 gms = 60 cals	2 gms = 8 cals	———
Fruit	10 gms = 40 cals	———	———
	37 gms = 148 cals	17 gms = 68 cals	5 gms = 45 cals
Luncheon:			
List 1 Veg.	6 gms = 24 cals	2 gms = 8 cals	———
List 2 Veg.	7 gms = 28 cals	2 gms = 8 cals	———
Meat	———	14 gms = 56 cals	10 gms = 90 cals
Bread	15 gms = 60 cals	2 gms = 8 cals	———
Fruit	20 gms = 80 cals	———	———
	48 gms = 192 cals	20 gms = 80 cals	10 gms = 90 cals
Dinner:			
List 1 Veg.	3 gms = 12 cals	1 gm = 4 cals	———
List 2 Veg.	7 gms = 28 cals	2 gms = 8 cals	———
Meat	———	14 gms = 56 cals	10 gms = 90 cals
Bread	15 gms = 60 cals	2 gms = 8 cals	———
Fruit	20 gms = 80 cals	———	———
	45 gms = 180 cals	19 gms = 76 cals	10 gms = 90 cals
Snack:			
Fruit	10 gms = 40 cals	———	———
TOTAL	140 gms = 560 cals	56 gms = 224 cals	25 gms = 225 cals

(*Total Calories:* 1,009)

According to the exchange system, you get:

    (A) One List 1 vegetable exchange,
    (B) One List 2 vegetable exchange,
    (C) One bread exchange,
    (D) Two meat exchanges, and
    (E) Two fruit exchanges.

In selecting from the menu, give yourself:

    (A) One appetizer,
    (B) One salad,
    (C) One entrée,
    (D) One bread exchange,
    (E) One vegetable, and
    (F) One dessert.

Snack: With the 1000 calorie level, you can permit yourself one piece of fruit as a snack sometime during the day. The best time for most people is probably just before going to bed.

The table on page 57 shows that you will be getting an excellent balance of protein, carbohydrate, and fat at every meal of the day. However, in viewing these tables based on the Exchange System, remember that the exchanges are always *approximate*.

The 1200-Calorie Level

If you have started your diet at 800 or 1000 calories, and are now graduating upward, the 1200-calorie level will seem like a veritable feast. At 1200 calories, you are getting all of the nutrients you need in your diet; if you are in good health, you should be able to continue losing weight at this level for some time.

The major differences between this and the other two levels are in the bread, milk, meat, and fat exchanges.

Breakfast: The recommended breakfast remains the same as it is for the 800- and 1000-calorie levels. (See page 144.) However, if you happen to like a big breakfast, you can look over your daily allowance of exchanges and shift some from lunch and dinner to breakfast. (Since lunch is 357 calories, and dinner is 492 calories, this should be easy to do.)

Lunch: The 1200-calorie level offers you 357 calories for lunch, hardly a "starvation diet." The daily menus break down roughly into:

    (A) Two List 1 vegetable exchanges,
    (B) One List 2 vegetable exchange,
    (C) Two meat exchanges,
    (D) One bread exchange,
    (E) One fat exchange, and
    (F) Two fruit exchanges,

with an additional 40 calories supplied either by an extra fruit exchange or by vegetable exchanges, depending upon the day and the menu.

On the menus, this breaks down into:

    (A) One appetizer,
    (B) One salad,
    (C) One entrée,
    (D) One vegetable, and
    (E) One dessert,

with a bread exchange and a fat exchange of your choice. (See Lists 4 and 6, pages 43 and 48.)

THE 1200-CALORIE LEVEL

Meal	Carbohydrate (47%)	Protein (23%)	Fat (30%)
Breakfast:			
Milk	12 gms = 48 cals	8 gms = 32 cals	————
Meat	————	7 gms = 28 cals	5 gms = 45 cals
Bread*	15 gms = 60 cals	2 gms = 8 cals	————
Fruit	10 gms = 40 cals	————	————
	37 gms = 148 cals	17 gms = 68 cals	5 gms = 45 cals
Luncheon:			
List 1 Veg.	6 gms = 24 cals	2 gms = 8 cals	————
List 2 Veg.	7 gms = 28 cals	2 gms = 8 cals	————
Meat	————	14 gms = 56 cals	10 gms = 90 cals
Bread	15 gms = 60 cals	2 gms = 8 cals	————
Fat	————	————	5 gms = 45 cals
Fruit	20 gms = 80 cals	————	————
	48 gms = 142 cals	20 gms = 80 cals	15 gms = 135 cals
Dinner:			
List 1 Veg.	3 gms = 12 cals	1 gm = 4 cals	————
List 2 Veg.	7 gms = 28 cals	2 gms = 8 cals	————
Meat	————	28 gms = 112 cals	20 gms = 180 cals
Bread	15 gms = 60 cals	2 gms = 8 cals	————
Fruit	20 gms = 80 cals	————	————
	45 gms = 180 cals	33 gms = 132 cals	20 gms = 180 cals
Snack:			
Fruit	10 gms = 40 cals	————	————
TOTAL	140 gms = 560 cals	70 gms = 280 cals	40 gms = 360 cals

(Total Calories: 1200)

*If you wish to have butter with your bread at breakfast, substitute one fat exchange for half of your skim milk exchange.

Dinner: The dinner at the 1200-calorie level offers you 492 calories, divided among:

    (A) One List 1 vegetable exchange,
    (B) One List 2 vegetable exchange,
    (C) Four meat exchanges,
    (D) One bread exchange, and
    (E) Two fruit exchanges.

Admittedly, with the sudden jump to four meat exchanges, this does give you a large percentage of fat. However, as I have indicated earlier, the average American likes to have meat as the center of his or her meal; and this level does permit you to have — for example — a 4-ounce steak.

The exchanges here translate roughly into:

(A) One appetizer,
(B) One salad,
(C) A double entrée,
(D) One vegetable, and
(E) One dessert,

allowing for one bread exchange to accompany your meal.

Snack: At the 1200-calorie level, you can have a snack of one piece of fruit, perferably in the evening before going to bed.

To see how your balance of protein, carbohydrate, and fat relates to the three meals of the day, look over the table on page 59. Again, remember that the Exchange System is only an approximation of calories. Perhaps the thing that this table best exemplifies is how much your fat level increases with the increase in the meat exchange.

Achieving Your Maintenance Level

One of the biggest problems with most weight-reduction diets is that, as soon as you go off the diet, you gain the weight back because your body rapidly has to restore the nutrition it has lost. One of the objects of this plan is to see that your body gets its proper nutrition so that you do not have to eat to restore the balance. Another object to educate you so that by the time you have lost the weight you want to lose, you will know enough about your body and about nutrition to be able to eat sensibly. When you prepare a meal or go out to a restaurant, you will know precisely what you are eating and why.

When you have reached your proper weight, it is time to go back to the calculations described in Chapter 4 (see page 34), to find the number of calories you require in your daily diet. For example, let us say that you are 25 years old, your weight is 150 pounds, and you are mildly active. Your maintenance calorie level is 1950 calories per day. Within that amount, you are going to have to determine an adequate and balanced diet of protein, carbohydrate, and fat. If you do not, you will gain weight again.

Try to keep your intake of protein between 50 and 65 grams a day. (If you are an extremely active male, you may be able to use up to 70 grams of protein.) Keep your fats, particularly saturated fats, as low as you possibly can. Allow the largest percentage of your diet to be taken up by carbohydrates.

Perhaps most important, go back to the Exchange System and determine just how much of each exchange is right for you in a day — or even in a specific meal. (And be aware that, when you exceed your allowance, you will have to work off the excess with exercise or extra activity.)

To help you stick to your allowance, it might be helpful to fill in your allowances on the following list and keep it with you.

Breakfast

_____ Fruit exchanges, List 3
_____ Meat exchanges, List 5
_____ Bread exchanges, List 4
_____ Milk exchanges, List 7 or 8
_____ Fat exchanges, List 6
_____ Plain coffee or tea
_____ Total calories

Luncheon

_____ Meat exchanges, List 5
_____ Bread exchanges, List 4
_____ Vegetable exchanges, List 1
_____ Vegetable exchanges, List 2
_____ Fruit exchanges, List 3
_____ Milk exchanges, List 7 or 8
_____ Fat exchanges, List 6
_____ Plain coffee or tea
_____ Total calories

Dinner

_____ Meat exchanges, List 5
_____ Bread exchanges, List 4
_____ Vegetable exchanges, List 1
_____ Vegetable exchanges, List 2
_____ Fruit exchanges, List 3
_____ Fat exchanges, List 6
_____ Milk exchanges, List 7 or 8
_____ Plain coffee or tea
_____ Total calories

Between Meals

A.M. _____ Exchange
_____ Exchange
P.M. _____ Exchange
_____ Exchange
Evening _____ Exchange
_____ Exchange
_____ Exchange
_____ Total Calories

Inevitably, there will be times when you will slip and eat too much; it happens with everyone. However, the sooner you catch yourself and get back to the correct nutrition, the better off you will be. Estimate how much you have overeaten, and apportion the excess into the next twenty meals.

It is relatively easy to keep track of how many calories you are eating when you are preparing food at home. It is much more difficult to lose or maintain weight when someone else is preparing the food for you — especially if it is a restaurant chef who is less concerned with how he is nourishing you than with how he is teasing your palate.

Chapter 7

DINING OUT

The critical moment for one who is "on a diet" usually arrives when it becomes necessary to dine out — either at a restaurant or in someone's home. The inability to cope with a restaurant menu, or the reluctance to appear ungracious to a host or hostess, can be the complete undoing of your best intentions. However, there are ways of getting through these critical moments without discomfort or embarrassment, while staying within your calorie limitations and having an enjoyable time.

Getting through a dinner party is entirely dependent upon your ability to be frank and honest with your host or hostess well in advance of the evening. However, in getting through a restaurant menu, you are entirely on your own. If you learn a few simple rules, you can do it gracefully.

Rules for Dining Out

The most important rule in dining in a restaurant is always to order à la carte; do not order the dinners. It may not be as economical, but you can be sure of getting precisely what you want, the way you want it.

There are two other important factors to consider when eating in a restaurant. The first consideration is portion control — managing to eat only the amount you need — and the second is avoiding the addition of sauces, dressings, and fats to any dish. If you remember these two factors, making your selections should be relatively easy.

SELECTING AN ENTRÉE

When you scan the list of entrées on the menu of a fine restaurant, everything looks rich, enticing — and fattening. What you have to do is to "read between the lines," and you will find a great many entrées that you *can* order. The only thing that you should exclude entirely is food that is breaded and fried.

Of course the easiest selections to make are those that are broiled — for example, broiled lamb chops or chicken. (With the lamb chops, you do not eat the fat. When chicken is broiled, most of the fat drips away, but you may want to remove the skin, especially from the breast.) And you can almost always eat fish. If it comes in a special sauce — for example, if it is brook trout amandine — you simply ask for it to be served without the almond sauce. In a fine restaurant, the sauce is almost always added to the dish just before it is served. However, watch out for the word *sauté* on the menu. For example, salmon steak sauté meunière would mean that the salmon is cooked *in* the meunière sauce.

You can easily order lobster or steak and ask that butter or butter sauce not be added. With lobster, you may have to be emphatic to get your way. Chefs cannot seem to resist the temptation to pour butter over lobster. (One lady I know is in the habit of going back to the restaurant kitchen to make sure her lobster is prepared the way she wants it.)

Some people are compulsive members of the "Clean Plate Club." Their parents drummed it into their heads that it was a shame to waste food, because children somewhere else in the world were starving; so they learned never to leave a speck of food on their plates. This habit becomes particularly dangerous when you are served a steak that weighs from 14 to 18 ounces. If you do not know when to stop eating and call for the "doggie bag," ask the waiter to cut the steak in half *before* serving it, and to wrap up the other half for you to take home.

And finally, do not reach for the salt shaker as soon as your dish is served. Inevitably some salt will be added in cooking, and you really do not need more. You may not have to ask that your food not be salted in the kitchen, however, since the excess generally comes in the butter that is added to the dish.

SALAD

A salad of mixed greens or sliced tomatoes is a delightful addition to any meal. The most important consideration in ordering your salad is the dressing. The rule is: The thinner the dressing, the better off you are. Straight oil and vinegar is, of course, the thinnest and the lowest in calories. The thicker dressings are made with mayonnaise or sour cream, both of which are extremely high in calories (see pages 47–48).

In some restaurants, you can now make your own salad at a salad bar. You can easily make an entire meal of the salad, with all sorts of ingredients — including hard-boiled eggs, cheese, bean sprouts, and chick peas. You would, of course, choose oil and vinegar as your dressing and, if you want to keep the calorie level down as much as possible, pass up the olives and bacon bits.

VEGETABLES

In good restaurants, you can usually get vegetables served to you without a butter sauce. That is the major consideration for you in selecting your vegetables. A fine restaurant can generally anticipate its flow of customers and prepare vegetables in small batches so they do not have to sit in a steam pan for two hours getting soggy. The butter sauce, then, is applied just before they are served.

However, you should ask the waiter how vegetables are prepared in the specific restaurant. Because butter (or fat) will keep meat and vegetables relatively fresh, some restaurants do make the vegetables in advance and let them sit in butter sauce.

While there are a few limitations (you might not enjoy an artichoke without a sauce to dip it in), you can order and enjoy most restaurant vegetables without worrying too much about calories.

CONSIDER THE POTATO

The potato is a much maligned food. As with bread, most people consider it to be terribly fattening. But the potato is an excellent food, filled with nutrients, and it is not really that high in calories. The calories are in what we add to the poor, defenseless potato.

The potato listed in the bread exchange is 100 grams, or approximately 3½ ounces, for 68 calories. That is not extremely high. Even the average baked potato served in a gourmet restaurant (about 8 ounces, or 250 grams) comes to only 160 calories. Considering the nutrition you are getting along with the calories, that is very good.

However, most people do not eat the potato as it is: they place a couple of tablespoons of sour cream on top, for about 45 calories; two pats of butter, for 90 calories; a teaspoon of bacon bits (equal to about 1½ slices of bacon), for 70 calories; and possibly even a spoonful or so of grated cheese, for 30 calories. This additional 235 calories brings the value of the plain little baked potato up to a whopping 395 calories.

We may also have our potato whipped with 4 tablespoons of cream, for 90 calories, and a pat of butter, for 45 calories, making our 160-calorie potato worth 295 calories.

But the worst thing we do to the potato is to fry it in fat. An average restaurant serving of cottage fries comes to around 400 calories; and the average serving of french fries comes to around 450 to 480 calories.

So we should not blame the potato; it has 160 good calories to offer. It will very nicely fit into your "diet" as long as you have it baked and do not load it up with fat. You may also find that without all that butter, sour cream, and bacon you do not feel compelled to eat the whole thing.

DESSERTS

You don't have to say no to dessert, but you do have to be discriminating. Dessert doesn't have to be a rich chocolate mousse with lots of whipped cream on top. Many fine restaurants now offer fruit as dessert, or fruit and cheese. Perhaps most important, try to remember that you need not eat all of what is served to you.

Restaurant Calories

With time you can become a discriminating and knowledgeable diner. The great popularity of gourmet cooking in recent years has acquainted many people with how various special dishes are prepared. Learning the difference between home cooking and restaurant cooking can be just as important as being a gourmet in your own kitchen.

If you are in a business that requires you to attend lunches, dinners, banquets, and cocktail parties, this knowledge is even more important than it is for the average person who dines out only occasionally.

It is worthwhile for anyone to study the menu tables that follow. They show the approximate number of calories in the average restaurant serving of most foods. For easy reference, they have been divided into breakfast and luncheon or dinner servings. There is also a list of the most popular snack foods, a list of sweets and desserts, and lists of beverages and alcoholic drinks.

BREAKFAST

The entrées on the breakfast menus of most restaurants fall into two categories: (1) the carbohydrate group, which includes toast, French toast, pancakes, sweet rolls and doughnuts; and (2) the foods that are cooked in butter or oil, such as fried eggs, omelets, bacon, and perhaps sausage.

The average pancake cooked without oil is about 100 calories. There are usually three pancakes to a serving, so you get 300 calories. When 4 tablespoons of syrup and three pats of butter are added to this, the total value becomes 670 calories. You will notice in the table of breakfast foods that two eggs poached or boiled are 146 calories, but when fried or scrambled in butter, they become 236 calories. Eggs Benedict are never much less than 700 calories a serving.

RESTAURANT BREAKFAST MENU

Food	Amount	Calories
Eggs, fried or scrambled in butter	2	236
Egg omelette, with butter and cream	3 eggs	350
Eggs Benedict	average serving	700
Eggs, poached or boiled, no butter	2	146
Broiled lean ham steak	6 oz., raw weight	292
Broiled fillet steak	6 oz., raw weight	292
Bacon, crisp	4 slices	180
Broiled Canadian bacon	4 slices	146
Sausage, pan fried	4 links	224
Toast	2 slices	136
Toast, buttered	2 slices	225
French toast,	1 thick slice	244
Pancake	4–5 in., each	75 to 135
Waffle	4–5 in., each	175
Sweet roll	medium size, each	270
Danish pastry	medium, each	300
Croissant, pastry	each	250 to 300
Doughnuts, cake, iced	each	300
Doughnuts, bread, sugared	each	200
Syrups	4 tbsp.	240
Jelly, jam, restaurant pkg. e. g.	1 tsp level	35
Butter or margarine	1 pat	45

The dry breakfast cereals so widely used by Americans lend themselves to a relatively nutritious breakfast when combined with milk or some of the milk products. Unfortunately, practically all of the breakfast cereals today have both sugar and salt added, so their caloric value is often double that of plain cereals.

LUNCHEON AND DINNER

Most of the dishes on the restaurant luncheon and dinner menu are ordered for dinner, but occasionally they are eaten for lunch. Heading this menu is plain broiled chicken. One-half of a broiler is about 4 ounces of protein. The reason for eating the chicken is that you want the protein. Four ounces equals 292 calories, but if the chef bastes it with butter in the cooking, you get another 90 calories and are now up to 382 calories. Down at the corner fast-food restaurant, you might order chicken that is cooked in deep fat under pressure. In this process, the fat is forced under pressure to the very bone of the chicken, so that the entire chicken is saturated with fat. Now the chicken becomes a serving of 580 calories — approximately 300 calories of protein and 300 of fat.

Further down in the list, you can see how much the addition of a rich sauce or gravy adds to a serving of beef, pork, lamb, chicken, or turkey. Also notice that the average TV dinner is approximately 550 calories. The addition of fat in any form, or the addition of butter or margarine even in small amounts, adds a tremendous amount of calories to any protein serving.

RESTAURANT LUNCHEON AND DINNER MENU

Food	Amount	Calories
Chicken, broiled, plain	½	292
basted with butter	½	382
roasted, deep fat, under pressure	½	580
New York strip steak, broiled	10 oz.	629
Broiled fillet, plain, no butter or sauce	8 oz.	438
Prime Rib au jus	large	730
Turkey, chicken, lamb, pork, or beef, roasted on a rack	6 oz. cooked weight	438
with rich sauce or gravy		600
TV Dinner	average	550
Spaghetti or ravioli with meat sauce		600
Lobster, steamed, plain	8 oz.	350
Lobster, broiled with butter	8 oz.	500
Dover Sole with butter	8 oz.	700
Salmon steak, broiled with butter	8 oz.	700
Caesar Salad	per serving	364
Hard "French roll"	1	136
Soft dinner roll	1 small	68
Liver paté	1 Tbsp. level	80

LUNCH AND SNACK FOODS

The first item on the table of popular lunch and snack foods is the low-calorie "businessman's" diet plate called a "low-calorie plate" in some restaurants. It usually contains 4 ounces of hamburger, a cup of cottage cheese, two slices of tomato, a slice of bread, and a gelatin dessert with whipped cream, for a grand total of 650 to 750 calories.

RESTAURANT LUNCH AND SNACK FOODS

Food	Amount	Calories
Low-calorie businessman's diet plate		650 to 750
English muffin, buttered		225 to 250
Chef's salad bowl;		
meat, egg, cheese, turkey	4 oz.	
greens	large bowl	
oil and vinegar dressing	2 Tbsp	432
with mayonnaise or sour		
cream dressing	4 oz.	881
Cracked Dungeness crab	1 crab	529
with red cocktail sauce		589
with mustard-mayonnaise		978
Thick soup	bowl	300
Medium thick soup	bowl	136
(6 oz. cup = ½ bowl)		
Club sandwich	3 slices bread	600
Ruben sandwich		1100
Monte Cristo, sautéed in butter		960
Chicken salad or egg salad sandwich	average	510
Meat, chicken, or turkey	3 oz. cooked weight	
sandwich with all the trimmings		512
Meat sandwich, chicken or turkey, with no		
butter or mayonnaise	3 oz.	370
Hamburger with all trimmings	4 oz.	500
without butter, mayonnaise, sweet relish,		
onion		370
Cheeseburger with all trimmings		580
without butter, mayonnaise, sweet relish,		
onion		443
Swiss cheese on rye bread with mayonnaise,		
butter, and mustard		450
without mayonnaise or butter		350
Grilled cheese sandwich, fried in butter		500
Toasted cheese sandwich, no mayonnaise		
or butter		285
"Hot dog" sandwich; frankfurter, bun,		
relish, mustard, mayonnaise		325
with mustard only		220
Slaw as served with sandwiches	1 scoop	60
Potato salad as served with sandwiches		250
Pizza with cheese, pepperoni, etc.	14-in. pie	1440
Pizza (⅛ × 14-in. pie)	5½" wedge	180
Chili	bowl	500 to 600
Cold salmon plate with lettuce, onion,		
tomatoes, red cocktail sauce or lemon		
(no mayonnaise)	3 oz. salmon	300
Shrimp bowl or double shrimp cocktail,		
red cocktail sauce or lemon	8 shrimp, large	250
Cheese, av. 17 varieties	1 oz.	100
Bologna or salami	2 thin slices, 1 oz.	100

Lunch and Snack Foods (Cont.)

Food	Amount	Calories
Nuts, shelled, dry roasted	4 oz.	200
roasted in oil		300
Hors d' oeuvre, av.	each	100
Potato chips	each	11
French fried potatoes	each	16
Olives	1 large	15
Pickles	1 dill, 1 tsp. relish, or 3 slices sweet pickle	30
Pretzels	1 medium	20
Popcorn, dry	1 cup loose packed	35
Popcorn, buttered	1 cup loose packed	80
Herring in sour cream	2 oz. serving	120

A small steak, a salad with oil and vinegar, and a piece of fruit provide a much better balance and contain considerably fewer calories than this "low-calorie" plate.

Very likely, many of your favorite foods can be found on this list. Note that a sandwich without butter or mayonnaise is almost as nutritious as it is with them — yet not using them can save you at least 100 calories. Fried sandwiches are relatively high in calories, at 500 to 1000 calories each. A grilled cheese sandwich, for instance, is fried in butter, giving it an approximate total of 500 calories, while a toasted cheese sandwich with no mayonnaise or butter is only 285.

You may be shocked to realize that each potato chip is 11 calories, and each french fried potato on our plate is 16 calories. Of course, these foods have a high fat content.

A friend of mine once came to La Costa to have lunch with me. Knowing my concern with nutrition, he wanted to show off his intelligent approach to food; when his order was taken, he loudly asked the waitress to bring him a hamburger patty with no bun. I'm sure that everyone at the table was very impressed with his dietary discrimination; however, I noticed that when his hamburger arrived without the bun, there was a pile of french fries on the side of his plate. Out of the corner of my eye, I counted thirty-five fries, and my friend ate every one of them. Calorically speaking, he would have benefitted more if he had ordered the hamburger patty with 2½ buns and declined the potatoes fried in deep fat — and he would have received more nourishment.

SWEETS AND DESSERTS

Sweets and pastries are well known to be high-calorie foods. Ice creams, candies, sundaes, deluxe milkshakes, layer cakes, pies, cookies, doughnuts, and sweet rolls are not only high in carbohydrate, but some of them contain large amounts of fat. Many of the foods in the table of sweets and desserts are psychologically habit-forming. It is not that your body needs these foods, but that by habit you feel you won't be happy unless you have a rich treat. Next time you are tempted, ask yourself if these high-fat and high-sugar foods are really worth what you are paying for them physiologically.

RESTAURANT SWEETS AND DESSERTS

Food	Amount	Calories
Ice cream	1 dip	100
with small cone		35
à la mode for cake or pie		158
	1 large scoop	275 to 350
Sherbet	restaurant serving	220 to 240
Chocolate sauce	2 tbsp. level	100
Ice cream soda	fountain size	290
Ice cream sundae; with ice cream, nuts, cherry, syrup, whipped cream	average	450
Chocolate milkshake	deluxe	800
made with ice milk		500
pre-mix, frozen		340
Peach Melba deluxe	restaurant serving	600
Cherries Jubilee	restaurant, flamed	600
Yogurt, plain	8 oz. (1 cup)	170 to 200
Yogurt, fruit flavored with sugar		240
Cookies and cake:		
Assorted cookies	each	100
Meringue drop cookies	each	35
Almond macaroons	each	50
Pound cake or plain, uniced loaf cake	½ in. slice	250
Layer cake, iced	average	450
Cupcake, iced	each	350
Sponge cake	av. slice	115
iced	av. slice	175
Pie	av. slice	350
Macedoine of fruit with sugar and brandy	restaurant serving	350
Jell-O, sugar, artificial flavoring	large sundae glass	150
with whipped cream		250
Candy:		
Chocolate cream or bon bon	large	200 to 365
Chocolate-covered mints	1 oz.	150
Hard candies	1 oz.	110
Jellied candies, gum drops, fruit, licorice	1 oz.	100
Marshmallows	1 oz.	100
chocolate coated	1 oz.	122
Solid choolate for baking, bitter	1 oz.	169
sweet	1 oz.	150
Caramels	1 oz.	120
Chocolate-coated candy bar	average	250
Pure milk chocolate bar	1 oz.	146
Almond bar, chocolate	1 oz.	155
Chocolate-coated coconut or caramel	1 oz.	130 to 150

Notice in the table that one large chocolate cream or bon bon can be as much as 365 calories. It is so easy to reach into a box of candy three or four times in an evening while watching television, especially if you have formed the dangerous habit of craving sweets at that time of day, every day. But it may be less easy if you remember that you are reaching for 1095 to 1460 calories. When you realize that you can enjoy a luncheon of 3 ounces of meat, a salad, a vegetable, and a dessert of fruit for the same number of calories that is found in one piece of pound cake, you should have no problem in choosing the proper food.

BEVERAGES

Americans as a whole consume enormous quantities of beverages, both nonalcoholic and alcoholic. For convenience, we have divided these beverages into two separate tables.

We all seem to forget that the finest beverage we can consume is water. As I have indicated in Chapter 3, you can get water from a variety of sources, including coffee and tea. Without cream or sugar, these beverages contain practically no calories. The caffeine in coffee disturbs some people because of its stimulating effect, but some of the decaffeinated varieties are quite acceptable. Herb teas, an excellent substitute for regular tea, offer both pleasant taste and variety.

BEVERAGES

Kind	Amount	Calories
Coffee or tea	as desired	negligible
Milk, whole	8 oz.	170
Milk, 2%	8 oz.	125
Milk, 1%	8 oz.	100
Milk, nonfat (skim)*	8 oz.	80
Hot cocoa, all milk with whipped cream		370
Hot cocoa pre-mix, no whipped cream		116
Orange juice, restaurant serving containing sugar	6 oz.	96
Tomato juice	6 oz.	45
Bottled soft drinks, such as colas and other carbonated drinks with sugar	8 oz. glass	96 to 100
	12 oz. bottle	av. 150
Ginger Ale	8 oz. glass	85
	12 oz. bottle	130
Low-calorie drinks, no sugar used	8–12 oz.	negligible
Chocolate milk drink	8 oz. av.	200

If milk is fortified with milk solids, add 15 to 20 calories.

Milk has been discussed under the milk exchanges in Chapter 5, but you should be reminded that whole milk contains approximately 4 percent fat. Low-fat milk contains approximately 2 percent fat, and nonfat, or skim, milk has a very small percentage of fat. One percent milk is often advertised as "99 percent fat free." The words *fat free* often used in advertisements seem to have a magical effect on people who are struggling to keep their weight down. Milk is an important food, and one of the best sources of calcium. If you feel that you cannot tolerate nonfat milk, the one percent milk can be substituted, as long as you realize that "fat free" does not mean "calorie free."

It is widely held by nutritionists that adults and children over one year of age, should never consume whole milk unless there is a medical indication for it. You can see in the beverage table the difference between the caloric content of hot cocoa made with milk and of whipped cream and the pre-mix cocoa made with skim milk and without whipped cream. Most restaurants serve a pre-mix hot chocolate that comes in package form and is made by adding water.

Juices are discussed under the fruit exchanges in Chapter 5. Restaurants often serve juices made from concentrate with sugar added. To know exactly the number of calories in the juice you are drinking, read the juice container label carefully or ask your waiter.

Most bottled drinks that contain sugar will average close to 100 calories for every 8-ounce glass. The low-calorie drinks list the number of calories per 8- or 12-ounce serving on the label of the can or bottle. Many of the low-calorie cola drinks contain caffeine, and it has been reported that they can be habit-forming. There are other low-calorie drinks that are thirst-quenching and pleasant and contain only one or two calories per 8-ounce serving. Try to avoid those that contain caffeine or salt, and remember that calories consumed in this manner are usually considered empty calories.

ALCOHOLIC BEVERAGES

A recent Gallup Poll indicates that 71 percent of Americans over eighteen drink beer, wine, or liquor — an all-time high (in more ways than one!). While very small amounts of alcohol may increase the appetite, it has been well established that large amounts definitely suppress the appetite. Alcohol is very high in calories and its consumption should certainly be limited when one is attempting to maintain or lose weight.

In determining the caloric content of alcoholic beverages, a general rule is that an alcoholic beverage contains approximately one calorie per proof per

ALCOHOLIC BEVERAGES

Kind	Average serving	Calories
Beer	12 oz.	150-185
Dry wines		
22 proof, white	1 oz.	22
24 proof, red	1 oz.	24
30 proof, sherry	1 oz.	30
Dessert wine, red, white, and port	1 oz.	45
Whiskey, rye, bourbon, rum, and brandy, 100 proof	1 oz.	100
Champagne, domestic	4 oz.	85
Gin and Scotch, 86 proof	1 oz.	86
Liqueurs, average	1 oz.	100
Mixed drinks		
Martini	standard	140
Manhattan	standard	165
Old-fashioned	4 oz.	180
Daiquiri	3½ oz.	125
Egg nog	4 oz.	335

ounce if it is plain and unfortified. For example, one ounce of 90 proof whiskey or vodka yields approximately 90 calories. If mixtures are used, or if other carbohydrates, such as sugar or malt, are present, the caloric value rises accordingly. In the average bar, a serving is approximately 1½ ounces. In the home, the average serving is usually 2 ounces. Cocktails with the addition of sugar and fruit juices — daiquiris, old-fashioneds, screwdrivers — have a considerably higher caloric value.

An excellent way to cut down on alcohol, and still be able to attend a cocktail party or sit in a bar with your friends, is to have dry wine instead of liquor. Many excellent dry wines can be found with 22 or 24 proof, so it is possible to have a large goblet of approximately 4 ounces of wine in exchange for one ounce of whiskey, gin, or vodka.

However, you should still remember that wine does have some calories, even though it has fewer than the stronger drinks. I recall a guest who came to my house one Christmas Eve for a drink and declared that she was "cutting down on her calories" by drinking only wine. In honor of the holiday, I brought out some of my best wine — and she proceeded to drink a bottle and a half of it!

Up until a few years ago, only heavy drinkers drank before 5 P.M., but today, business breakfasts often begin with a screwdriver or a Bloody Mary, and business luncheons with a round of martinis. Many people don't realize that alcohol is almost a pure carbohydrate. They will sit and consume 500, 600, or even 1000 calories of pure carbohydrate in drinks at a bar or at a party. Then, when they are ushered in to dinner, they push back a 160-calorie potato or a slice of bread and announce loudly that they never eat carbohydrates. Anyone who dines this way both gains weight and starves his body for fats, proteins, and vitamins, thus inviting any number of deficiency diseases.

It is important to know that the body, in its metabolic processes, does not treat alcohol as a carbohydrate. If the alcohol taken in is not burned up immediately, it is deposited directly into the body as fat.

Of course, you cannot learn a great deal about food and beverages simply by dining out in restaurants. The place to find out about food is your local "food library" — your supermarket. Some of the most valuable information you can gain is on the labels of cans and bottles. True, some of them may seem at first to be written in a foreign language, but once you learn the technique of reading them, it becomes easy.

Chapter 8

SHOPPING

Nutritional Labeling

The average supermarket today contains approximately ten thousand different products, over half of which are packaged foods. These are now subject to the requirement or "nutritional labeling" that has been developed by the Food and Drug Administration to correct and act against false labeling or deceptive promotion of products. The aim of the new labeling is to give shoppers a better knowledge of what they are buying.

The FDA regulations also require full and honest labeling of vitamin and mineral products, whether they are sold as foods, as dietary supplements, or as drugs. These regulations seek to protect the consumer against the promotional claims made for certain dietary supplements that are so low in potency that they are not effective nutritionally, or so high that they exceed any reasonable definition of a dietary supplement.

The abbreviation "U.S. RDA" stands for United States Recommended Daily Allowances. These recommended allowances were determined after years of study and were published by the Food and Nutrition Board of the National Academy of Sciences, and recommended by the National Research Council. The U.S. RDA represents the quantity of nutrients needed every day by healthy people, allowing an excess of 30 to 50 percent for individual variations. Any product containing more than 150 percent of the U.S. RDA is considered a drug. To protect the consumer, such products will be regulated by the FDA and marketed by industry as drugs.

Nutritional labeling is not yet found on every packaged food, but within the next few years most of the foods will have it, so that the consumer can compare products and find the one that gives him the most nutrition or that fits his individual program. The first part of each label is a statement of "Nutrition Information." It tells the size of the serving, the number of servings in the container, and the number of calories and the amounts of protein, carbohydrate, and fat in each serving. The second part of the label lists the percentages of the U.S. Recommended Daily Allowances of protein, vitamins, and minerals found in that product. A typical nutrition information label may look like this:

SWEET PEAS

Net Wt. . . . . 8½ oz. or 241 grams   Cups Approx. 1

INGREDIENTS: PEAS, WATER, SUGAR, SALT

NUTRITION INFORMATION — PER ONE CUP PORTION

CALORIES 105   FAT . . . . .1 gm
PROTEIN . . . . .7 gm   CARBOHYDRATE (avail.) . . .16 gms

PERCENTAGE OF U.S. RECOMMENDED DAILY ALLOWANCE (U.S. RDA)
    PER ONE CUP PORTION

PROTEIN .10   NIACIN 8
VITAMIN A 20   CALCIUM 2
VITAMIN C 35   IRON 10
THIAMIN (B₁) 10   PHOSPHORUS 10
RIBROFLAVIN (B₂) 8   MAGNESIUM 6

The following tables show (1) nutrients in the order in which they must appear on nutrition labels, and (2) the order and the amounts in which vitamin and mineral supplements are recommended according to the U.S. RDA.

U.S. RECOMMENDED DAILY ALLOWANCE FOR ADULTS AND CHILDREN OVER 4 YEARS (U.S. RDA)

Vitamins and Minerals	*Quantity*
PROTEIN	65 gm*
VITAMIN A	5,000 IU*
VITAMIN C	60 mg*
THIAMINE	1.5 mg
RIBOFLAVIN	1.7 mg
NIACIN	20 mg
CALCIUM	1.0 gm
IRON	18 mg
VITAMIN D	400 IU*
VITAMIN E	30 IU*
VITAMIN B₆	2.0 mg
FOLICIN	0.4 mg
VITAMIN B₁₂	6 mcg*
PHOSPHORUS	1.0 gm
IODINE	150 mcg
MAGNESIUM	400 mg
ZINC	15 mg
COPPER	2 mg
BIOTIN	0.3 mg
PANTOTHENIC ACID	10 mg

*gm = grams   *mg = milligrams
*IU = International Units   *mcg = micrograms

U.S. RECOMMENDED DAILY ALLOWANCES ADULTS AND CHILDREN 4 OR MORE YEARS OF AGE (U.S. RDA)
(FOR LABELING VITAMIN AND MINERAL SUPPLEMENTS)

Vitamins and Minerals	Quantity
VITAMIN A	5,000 IU
VITAMIN D	400 IU
VITAMIN E	30 IU
VITAMIN C	60 mg
FOLIC ACID	0.4 mg
THIAMINE	1.5 mg
RIBOFLAVIN	1.7 mg
NIACIN	20 mg
VITAMIN B_6	2.0 mg
VITAMIN B_{12}	6 mcg
BIOTIN	0.3 mg
PANTOTHENIC ACID	10 mg
CALCIUM	1.0 gm
PHOSPHORUS	1.0 gm
IODINE	150 mcg
IRON	18 mg
MAGNESIUM	400 mg
COPPER	2.0 mg
ZINC	15 mg

To be wise and efficient shoppers, we should all read the nutrition information listed on packaged foods. It will aid us in providing ourselves and our families with an adequate, well-balanced, and healthful diet.

A Trip Through the Supermarket

When I was a boy, shopping was quite different from what it is today. I often accompanied my mother on her weekly shopping tour, and we always had to make a number of stops. For vegetables and fruits, we went to the greengrocer's. For meat, we went to the butcher shop, where we would watch the butcher cut the meat to the size and the specifications we had given him. Baked goods were always on our lists, which meant going to the bakery. A stop at the dairy was necessary to get our milk and milk products. Any other items we wanted could usually be found at the general store. Shopping in this manner was time consuming, and the transportation cost today would be prohibitive. Now our lives are geared to one-stop shopping. All of the food products we need can now be found under one large roof, with adequate parking and easy access.

Walking into a supermarket today, you cannot help being impressed not only by the size of the store, but also by the colorful displays, the wide variety of attractively packaged fresh foods, the convenient arrangements of these foods on the shelves, and the signs identifying the various departments to make it easy for the shopper to locate the items on his list. But you must realize that once you enter a supermarket, you are in the hands of a highly developed science known as merchandising.

The way the foods are presented to you, the backgrounds, the lighting and color schemes, have a great deal of influence on what you buy and on the amounts you purchase. If you happen to want a loaf of bread, a pound of butter, and a quart of milk, these "everyday" items are always placed as far away from the cash register as possible, so that in walking through the store to get these foods, you will see hundreds of other items available to you. The power of suggestion plays a tremendous part in selling you more than you really came to buy.

The average supermarket today contains well over ten thousand items; approximately 10 percent of these are not food items, such as magazines, tennis shoes, hardware, pet supplies, kitchen ware, antifreeze, laundry detergents, and paper goods. The food products in a supermarket can be found in almost any form — fresh, raw, frozen, dehydrated, ground, cooked in various combinations or with sauces, and packaged in different ways and amounts. The merchandiser in a supermarket knows that the prime selling area on a shelf is between the top of your head and your waist, so that you are looking directly at the product he wants you to buy. This is the area in which the higher-priced foods are placed. The cheaper foods are usually found on the lower shelves, or on the extremely high shelves. Naturally, you are attracted to the items that are directly in your line of sight and within easy reach.

T. W. Feed, in *Food Merchandising* (1973), made a study of consumer buying habits and found that when food products were moved from waist level to eye level, sales increased by almost 37 percent. The moving of these same products to floor level caused the sales to fall off by over 70 percent.

As you enter a beautiful, brightly lit supermarket, you usually find carts conveniently located near the entrance door. After taking your cart, if you are right-handed like most people, you automatically turn to the left. In many markets the first thing you see is a glorious arrangement of plants in season, such as poinsettias at Christmas, or fall chrysanthemums, or daffodils in the spring. It is hard for the average person to resist these beautiful plants and they put you into a buying mood.

FRUITS AND VEGETABLES

At some point in your supermarket tour you come to a huge display of fruits and vegetables. These are exhibited in a way that hardly anyone can resist. The fruits and vegetables are colorful, clean, and somewhat aromatic, and have been brightly polished. The polish, especially on fruits such as apples and pears, as well as on vegetables such as cucumbers, does make a difference. A bin of polished apples located beside a bin of unpolished apples will outsell the unpolished apples almost ten to one. This polishing of fruits is done by a wax rinse, which is trivial in amount, and it coats the fruit to make it shine. It is also done to preserve the moisture and nutrient value of fruits that have been transported over great distances. In choosing fruits and vegetables, however, remember that they taste best and are most nutritious when they are in season. It is also better, where possible, to purchase local fruits and vegetables than those that have been shipped from a distant region, as the time it takes to transport them can cause a loss of flavor and nutritional value if they are unwaxed.

The preservative wax is harmless and can be removed by washing. It is wise never to wash and trim vegetables or fruits until you are ready to serve them. In planning a meal, prepare only the amount of fruits and vegetables that will be used for that meal. Produce should always be well shaped, crisp, and firm and should show no wrinkling of the skin and no wilting or brown ends. Of course, cook fruits and vegetables with their skin intact whenever possible. Many of the minerals and vitamins are stored in the area of the skin or hull. Also, remember that the darker or more deeply colored fruits and vegetables usually have the most nutritive value. Dark green lettuce, for example, is far more nutritious than the pale, light-colored variety. Remember to buy tomatoes that are deep red and carrots that are bright orange.

PACKAGED FOODS

When you come to the packaged foods in the supermarket, reading the labels is imperative if you are to understand what the product contains. According to U.S. labeling laws, all packaged foods and canned foods must list the ingredients in order of predominance. The first item is the largest by either volume or weight, and the subsequent items follow in the order of their amount in the product.

There are a number of packaged foods that do not list ingredients. These fall into the a category known as "standardized items," those that meet certain standards of identity set by federal regulations. The formulas for these foods are on file with the Food and Drug Administration, and unless there is some variation, the package merely states what the product is. For example, a label may state "Pure Strawberry Preserves," which means that it is made of strawberries and sugar in equal proportions. Another example is mayonnaise, which need not list ingredients as long as it does not vary from the standard formula of mayonnaise. A further example is ice cream. If it meets the standard of identity set up by the government, and if nothing is omitted or added, it requires only the label "Ice Cream."

If a product is artificially sweetened or colored, or contains other ingredients, these must be listed in the order of their predominance by either weight or volume. A label for imitation strawberry preserves, for example, might read: apple base, sugar, strawberries, artificially colored and flavored. If a product is called "Corned Beef Hash," it must have at least 35 percent beef and must contain potatoes, curing agents, and seasoning. It may contain onions, garlic, beef broth and beef fat, and so on, but it cannot contain more than 15 percent fat, and no more than 72 percent moisture.

The food value of two similar products can vary a great deal, so it is a good idea to take up the habit of reading the ingredients listed on the packages. A recent survey has shown that, although 90 percent of shoppers claim to understand nutritional labeling, only half of those making the claim actually know how to use the information, because most of it is presented in terms that are too technical. One thing is easy to tell, however: If the list is long and cumbersome, and you become confused by the ingredients, you can be certain that it has been altered or adulterated, or is an imitation product.

Everyone should be familiar with labeling, and if you are interested in becoming a more intelligent shopper, you can request a list of standardized items from the U.S. Department of Agriculture, Washington, D.C., 20250.

CONDIMENTS

Having filled your shopping basket with fruits, vegetables, and packaged goods, you move toward the back of the store. On your way, you pass the shelf of condiments. Included here are the meat sauces, ketchup, mustards, salt and salt substitutes, and of course, a large variety of spices.

Where spices are concerned, in addition to reading the ingredients carefully, you should notice the date stamped on the top or bottom of the container. The date on spices usually is the year it was packaged. The "shelf life" of spices — the period during which they remain effective — is about one year. After that, most spices lose their effectiveness, even if the package is sealed. Their aroma comes from the volatile oils and may last only a few weeks if the spices are kept in open bottles. Black pepper, which is used in almost every home and restaurant, can lose its effectiveness after a week of being exposed in pepper shakers. Check your spice rack at home frequently, because many of the spices found in open bottles have long since lost their flavor and aroma, and should be replaced by fresh spices.

Salt substitutes are one item that you should analyze by careful label reading. The most common substitute for the sodium ion found in table salt is potassium. Potassium is bitter, and many salt substitutes list potassium as the predominant ingredient. Sugar is often added to these salt substitutes to counteract the bitter potassium flavor. This addition enhances the taste remarkably, but it adds calories. Beware of the label that reads "Seasoned Salt Substitute." "Seasoned" allows the manufacturer to add any number of ingredients to the product, some of which may not be beneficial to you.

BAKERY

After the spices and condiments, the next big display that meets the eye may be the bakery section with the shelves of bread. If you are trying to lose weight, or at least to eat intelligently, the goodies found in these shelves — cookies, pies, cakes, sweet rolls, and so forth — should be passed by quickly.

One thing that can be confusing here is the varieties of bread. I have counted as many as twenty-five different types of bread in a supermarket. Contrary to popular belief, bread is not a high-calorie food. A slice of bread weighing 25 grams usually amounts to only about 68 calories. For the most part, choosing your favorite type of bread is not going to make a difference in calories per slice more than a few calories one way or the other. No one bread is any better for you than any other, and many of them are fortified with so many extras that they hardly resemble bread. Even some of the "natural" breads have additives. So again, label reading is most important. You do not want to buy breads that have highly caloric additions of molasses, fruits, or raisins.

DAIRY

After you have made your choices in the bakery section, you push your basket along the back wall of the supermarket. Here you find a fantastic display of dairy products. As you approach this section, you are subconsciously impressed by the pure white, spotlessly clean shelves of milk, butter, cheese, and yogurt.

Practically all of the dairy products found in the supermarket refrigerators have a date stamped on them. This is the shelf life date, and it is found usually on the handle of the milk carton, and on the top or bottom of the yogurt, cream, or sour cream carton. This date merely indicates that the product should be used by that time; following this date, the product may deteriorate. It does not mean that after this date, these products are of no value. It simply gives you a warning that you should use these products by that time, in order to get their full value.

Milk: Milk is an excellent food and an excellent source of protein as well as one of the few sources of calcium, and it often contains many other vitamins and minerals. It is one of the main sources of riboflavin. In certain forms, it can also supply considerable amounts of fat and sugar. As you stand in front of this display shelf, the different types of milks can be often confusing, so I will discuss each one separately.

Fresh Whole Milk: Whole milk in liquid form is usually found in cartons labeled "whole milk." Many brands today are fortified with both minerals and vitamins and most are homogenized. In homogenized milk, the milk fat globules have been broken down in size; therefore, the cream does not separate from the milk and the product stays relatively uniform. All milk must be pasteurized, and the rating "Grade A" designates wholesomeness rather than any level of quality.

The Public Health Service of whatever state the milk is purchased in usually has an ordinance that requires whole milk to have no less than 3.25 percent milk fat. It occasionally runs up to as high as 4 percent. To show how gullible most consumers are, an advertising firm once placed an ad in a magazine showing a beautiful glass of milk, stating that this milk was "96 percent fat free." Thousands of people wrote in to find out where they could buy this wonderful new milk preparation. Most people do not realize that this is whole milk — that whole milk *is* 96 percent fat free — nor do they realize that it contains 4 percent fat. The only difference between a glass of skim milk and a glass of whole milk is that an 8-ounce glass of whole milk contains the equivalent of two pats of butter.

Low-Fat Milk: Low-fat milk, which is occasionally called 2 percent milk, contains between 0.5 percent and 2 percent milk fat, depending on the regulations of the locality where it is purchased. If you mix whole milk and skim milk in equal parts, the result is a low-fat milk of approximately 2 percent milk fat.

One Percent Milk: In certain areas in the United States, milk is sold as one percent, or is occasionally labeled "99 percent fat free." This milk merely has one-fourth the butterfat of whole milk, or one-half the butterfat of 2 percent milk, but occasionally it is advertised as having 20 percent more protein. This is accomplished by adding milk solids, and the calories are naturally increased.

Skim Milk: Fresh skim milk, better known as non-fat milk, in most states has less than 0.5 percent milk fat. Of course, it too is often fortified with vitamins, especially A and D. Remember that skim milk has most of the nutrients that whole milk has, except for the fat and the fat-soluble vitamins.

Cream: If you are interested in losing weight and avoiding milk fat, you should pass up the creams in the dairy product section. The following is a list of the various percentages of fat found in the average creams.

Light Cream: This is often called "coffee" or "table" cream. According to federal standards of identity, it must have at least 18 percent milk fat.

Half-and-Half: Half-and-half is a mixture of milk and cream. Again, under the standards of identity, it must contain approximately 10 to 12 percent milk fat.

Light Whipping Cream: Whipping cream of all types has a high percentage of milk fat, and federal standards of identity require light whipping cream to have 30 percent milk fat.

Heavy Whipping Cream: Heavy whipping cream is somewhat heavier in milk fat than light whipping cream. The standard is approximately 36 percent.

Sour Cream: Sour cream is occasionally called "cream dressing" or "salad cream." It is made by adding lactic acid bacteria culture to a light cream. It contains approximately 18 percent milk fat.

Sour Half-and-Half: Sour half-and-half is the same as half-and-half, except that a culture has been added. It contains approximately 10 to 12 percent milk fat.

Butter and Margarine: Butter and conventional margarines have approximately the same caloric value. Butter is made from churning pasturized cream. According to federal law, it must have at least 80 percent milk fat. Today, in the United States, twice as much margarine is sold as butter.

Both butter and margarine are sold in one-pound, half-pound, and quarter-pound packages. You can also buy both products in an unsalted form, which is necessary for people who must keep down their sodium intake. Both products also can be purchased in a whipped form that is approximately half the normal weight.

Butter and conventional margarine are fairly standardized as to flavor. The flavor of other types of margarine — such as soft, whipped, diet, imitation, and liquid — varies from brand to brand.

Approximately one-fourth of an average American's fat consumption is in the use of butter and margarine. A pound of butter or a pound of margarine contains 3500 calories of fat. The diet margarines may contain as little as 1700 calories. This means that butter and margarine have approximately 100 calories per tablespoon. Diet margarines contain approximately 50 calories per tablespoon, but you cannot depend on this figure unless it is clearly stated on the label.

If you want to cut down on sodium, you must remember that a tablespoon of either butter or margarine contains approximately 140 milligrams of sodium. Fortunately, you can buy both unsalted butter and unsalted margarine, which are estimated to contain 3 to 5 milligrams of sodium per tablespoon.

As you face the supermarket shelf of table spreads, be sure you know which product best fits your specific needs. If you have any questions about this, your physician can help guide you in the proper choice.

Cheese: Cheese is an excellent food, but it is also a very concentrated food that is high in calories and usually contains a large amount of salt. If you are trying to keep down your intake of calories, you should use cheese in small quantities.

There are basically two types of cheese. One is a pure cheese, made of the casein curd together with mold and the aging process. The other type is called processed cheese and it has other ingredients added, so check the label — there may be some things in a processed cheese that do not fit into your diet plan.

The cheese department of most supermarkets offers a wide selection. Most of the cheeses come in one-pound packages, although some of the more flavorful types are in one-ounce foil-wrapped packages. In the last few years, merchants have found that cheese sells better in odd-shaped packages than it does in a simple, plainly wrapped package. Therefore, almost every supermarket will have a basket or container filled with all sorts of sizes and shapes of cheese. Cheese food and cheese spreads are other forms available — again, read the label.

It is difficult to determine at a glance the price that you are paying for the cheese unless you study the label and analyze the cost per ounce or per pound. In the average supermarket it is not possible to buy a wedge of cheese off a wheel as you could in the old days when a grocer would cut it to size. Your state university or the Dairy Council can furnish you a catalog of cheeses that will describe the wide variety. Cheese can be a delicacy, so choose a good quality that you enjoy, and consume it in moderation.

Yogurt: Yogurt generally is made of whole milk that has been pasteurized and homogenized, with a special culture added to give it a custardlike texture. Yogurt has the same nutritive factors in it as the milk from which it is made. It can also be made from skim milk, or from 2 percent or low-fat milk. It is advisable to read the labels of yogurts, as you may find that some brands are not a pure milk substance, but have been thickened with gelatin or dry milk solids. Yogurt is often artificially flavored and sweetened with sugar, and in many brands, fruit has been added, which naturally raises the caloric value from 170 calories per cup (8 ounces) to 240 if made from whole milk. The shelf life of yogurt can be as long as one month if it is kept cold but not frozen.

Frozen Desserts: Frozen desserts, found in the freezer cabinets of supermarkets, include ice cream of various kinds, ice milk, sherbet, ices, and ice cream bars. Ice cream varies widely in different areas, depending on whether it is sold interstate or made locally. As a rule, ice cream is made from cream, milk, sugar, flavorings, and occasionally gelatin and stabilizers. According to the U.S. Department of Agriculture, it must contain a minimum of 10 percent milk fat. French ice cream, which is also called frozen custard, is ice cream with egg yolks added. Of course, the caloric value rises with this addition.

Ice milk also varies according to the area. It is made from milk, stabilizers, flavorings, and sugar. According to the laws governing interstate commerce, it must contain between 2 and 7 percent milk fat. The soft ice cream that is sold at roadside stands more nearly resembles ice milk than it does ice cream.

Many people think that sherbet is made from water and not milk, and therefore is low in calories. Sherbet is made from milk, fruit or fruit juice, stabilizers, and sugars. It has approximately twice as much sugar as ordinary ice cream, and it varies in its milk fat content from 1 to 3 percent.

EGGS

Always buy eggs that are in a refrigerated area. If they have been federally examined and graded, there is a shield-shaped grade mark that indicates the quality at the time of grading. It does not matter whether you buy white or brown eggs, because the color of the shell does not affect the quality or the nutrient value of an egg.

Eggs come in four sizes, and most markets carry all four. They are as follows:

U.S. Small — 18 ounces per dozen
U.S. Medium — 21 ounces per dozen
U.S. Large — 24 ounces per dozen
U.S. Extra Large — 27 ounces per dozen

These are the classifications required by the federal government. However, most merchandisers add their own classifications — Grades B, A, AA. Though these may vary slightly from place to place, they generally correspond to the government classifications.

The larger the egg, the more appealing it usually is, expecially if it is Grade AA. In the present market, if the difference in price between the various sizes is not more than six cents per dozen, you can assume that the larger egg is the most economical. Grade B eggs are satisfactory if they are to be used as a mixture in cooked dishes. (The difference between Grade A and Grade B is in the appearance: the Grade B eggs are not as perfectly formed.)

MEAT

As you have progressed through the various departments of the supermarket, and are making your way back toward the checkout counter, the next big section is the meat display. It is seldom that we go to the market without stopping at the meat counter, because most meals at home are planned around the meat that is to be served.

No longer do the larger supermarkets have butchers who will wait on you individually. All of the meat is packaged in cellophane wrappers and labeled so that you know the type, origin, cut, weight, and price per pound.

Meat Grading: The United States Department of Agriculture (USDA) is interested in making sure that consumers get the quality of meat they expect and pay for, so it has a service known as "meat grading," which is paid for by the packers but is government-controlled. Beef, lamb, and veal are so graded; but pork, since it is fairly standard, does not need to be graded.

 USDA Prime has a tremendous amount of marbling. A large percentage of this meat is fat, which, of course, contributes to its tenderness and flavor. If you want to avoid fat, you have to throw much of the weight away after trimming, so it is an expensive item.

 USDA Choice is a high-quality meat, and has much less fat and less marbling than Prime. It is the one that is usually found in the better retail stores. It is also less expensive than prime.

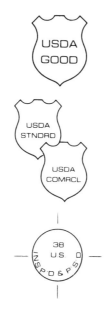

USDA Good has even less fat than Choice meat. It is just as nutritious as the other grades, but is considerably less expensive.

USDA Standard and USDA Commercial are seldom found in a supermarket. While they are almost as nutritious as the other grades, they are usually used only in the making of sausages.

You may occasionally run across a circle-shaped stamp as seen at the left, which shows that the meat is a processed product. It occasionally has other ingredients added, but it is a satisfactory product from the health standpoint. The contents of a processed product can be exceedingly varied.

The National Livestock and Meat Board has recently developed a meat identification code. It realizes that a single cut of meat is often labeled with as many as a dozen popular names, depending on where it is purchased. The Board has reduced from approximately 1,000 retail meat cuts to 300 standard names for fresh cuts of beef, veal, pork, and lamb. The customer has a right to know what he is buying and to know the value of the product in comparison to other cuts of meat. Therefore, the entire retail meat industry has agreed to establish one specific name for each basic retail cut. This all appears on the label.

Each piece of meat will have a meat department label, which gives the price of that particular piece, and the price per pound. Under the price, the first word is the origin of the meat, whether it is beef, pork, lamb, or veal. The second word is where the meat came from: chuck, rib, loin, round. Under this are words that describe the retail cut, whether it is a blade roast, spareribs, loin chops, and so on. This uniform identity labeling certainly takes the guesswork out of shopping; at a glance, you know exactly what you are buying.

Ground Beef: Ground beef is one of the most important items in the meat department. Until the new labeling system, it was often maligned because of its inconsistency. Now we no longer have an infinite number of variations in the quality of hamburger. The labeling on ground beef today follows the uniform retail meat identity standards code. Meat that is labeled "ground beef" must be pure beef, with no additions of variety meats or other ingredients. It is labeled in the percentage of lean, and there are usually three different degrees of label. This assures the customer exactly what he is getting in the package in the lean-fat ratio. The three classifications found in most stores are:

1. *Ground Beef:* Not less than 75 percent lean. This is the type of beef that we usually use in hamburgers, chili, and spaghetti sauce.

2. *Ground Beef:* Not less than 80 percent lean. This is the type of beef that is usually used in meat balls, meat loaf, and some of the beef and noodle or rice casseroles.

3. *Ground Beef:* Not less than 85 percent lean. This is the type that you should use in a low-calorie diet, as it is as lean as you can possibly buy.

Occasionally, a market may label its meat "Ground Beef, Chuck," "Ground Beef, Round," or "Ground Beef, Sirloin." However, the label still must specify the lean-to-fat ratio. When buying meat, be sure to pay attention to the date that the meat was wrapped. Choose the leanest meat you can, and buy only enough for one meal.

Today, there are a number of extenders being used with meat. The most common extender is texturized soy protein; occasionally you will see the letters "TSP" on a package of ground beef. This means that soybean has been used in a certain percentage to make the meat go further. Although meat with extenders is fairly economical, the use of extenders in too large an amount often impairs the flavor and texture of the meat.

The Care and Storage of Meats: Many people buy more meat than can be used by the family within the next day or two. If you freeze meat intending to keep it more than two weeks before using it, you should wrap it carefully in special freezer paper. Fresh meats should be used within two to three days. Ground meats and variety meats should always be used within 24 hours. The following chart, which was obtained from the U.S. Department of Agriculture, is a guide for both refrigerator and freezer storage.

MAXIMUM MEAT STORAGE TIME

Meat	*Refrigerator (36° to 40° F.)*	*Freezer (at 0°F or lower)*
Beef (fresh)	2 to 4 days	6 to 12 months
Veal (fresh)	2 to 4 days	6 to 9 months
Pork (fresh)	2 to 4 days	3 to 6 months
Lamb (fresh)	2 to 4 days	6 to 9 months
Ground beef, veal, and lamb	1 to 2 days	3 to 4 months
Ground pork	1 to 2 days	1 to 3 months
Variety meats	1 to 2 days	3 to 4 months
Luncheon meats	1 week	not recommended
Sausage, fresh pork	1 week	60 days
Sausage, smoked	3 to 7 days	
Sausage, dry and semi-dry (unsliced)	2 to 3 weeks	not recommended
Frankfurters	4 to 5 days	1 month
Bacon	5 to 7 days	1 month
Smoked ham, whole	1 week	60 days
Ham slices	3 to 4 days	60 days
Beef, corned	1 week	2 weeks
Leftover cooked meat	4 to 5 days	2 to 3 months

"DIETETIC" FOODS

As you leave the meat department and move toward the checkout area, you might suddenly decide to try one of the "dietetic" foods, perhaps canned peas prepared without sugar or salt, or a low-calorie salad dressing.

There is nothing magical about the word *dietetic;* it does not mean that a food so called has any protective value or is therapeutic or any better for you than ordinary foods in the proper amounts. Here again, it is very wise to read labels.

As you look at the signs that guide you to the items in the store, you may discover that the dietetic foods are located toward the middle; this is done for a purpose. It is interesting to note that in the majority of supermarkets, the dietetic and low-calorie foods are placed on a shelf over the freezer cabinet. As you reach up and over the cabinet to obtain the low-calorie item you want, you will probably glance down into the freezer, where some of the highest-calorie foods in the entire store are located. Here you find the frozen pizza, pies, and cakes, gourmet ice creams, and so forth. These beautiful displays of rich foods are very hard to resist, and seldom does one have the will power to ignore them. Most of us rationalize about the convenience of having at least one or two of these items on hand in the freezer for unexpected company.

THE CHECKOUT STAND

By the time you finally make your way toward the checkout area, you have made a complete tour of the store. You have been up many of the aisles to pick up the items you originally came to purchase. You have been in the middle of the store for dietetic foods and some of the high-calorie goodies, and have picked up many items that were not on your shopping list and that are probably not necessary. As you return to the front of the store, you have to pass the end displays on each aisle. These end displays are among the prime selling areas in the store. "Specials" are often put there, even though they do not always have a special price. Since they are so prominently displayed, your attention is drawn to each "special" as you walk toward the checker, and you are again tempted.

You may have noticed that there are usually at least two or three people ahead of you at the checkout counter; seldom do you find a counter where you can move your basket in immediately. As a result, you find yourself studying the counter displays of candies, mints, magazines, fad diet books, cigarettes, and assorted trinkets. Since you have a few minutes to wait, you will probably pick up one or two of these products.

You finally have your turn at the checkers. After you get the final total, and the food is bagged and ready to be transported to your car, you may be appalled that you have purchased a lot more than you had intended when you first came into the store. As you wheel your sacks of groceries out to your car, pull out the list of foods you had meant to buy, and have a good laugh at yourself for being enticed into buying so much. Maybe you will be more disciplined next time.

PART III

THE 14-MINUTE EXERCISE PLAN

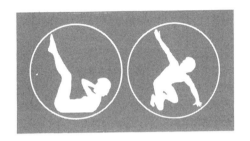

Chapter 9

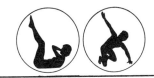

THE MINIMUM DAILY REQUIREMENT

A good diet for weight loss should always be accompanied by a program of exercise. Although the exercises in this chapter will not burn up a great many calories, they will help to keep you firm and trim and fit. One of the reasons you are dieting in the first place is that you want to improve the way you look and feel; and to do that, you are going to have to become reacquainted with your body.

These exercises will not take very much time out of your day. Although you will be given many exercises to choose from, you don't have to do all of them, and you don't have to spend much time with the ones that you do — only about 14 minutes a day.

However, if you sincerly wish to stay fit, you cannot stop exercising at the end of your 14-day diet. You will have to keep exercising at least 14 minutes a day for the rest of your life. In fact, one of your problems is that you stopped exercising somewhere along the line.

You Do Not Have To Sweat To Keep Fit

Admittedly, exercise is something that just about everybody hates. It is one habit we do not take to readily, because we are not brought up in a pattern that incorporates it as an enjoyable part of our daily lives. Instead, we have been made to feel that it is unpleasant or even painful. It is something we were forced to do back in high school physical education class or in military service. And, of course, that regimen was imposed upon us by someone disgustingly fit, possibly even muscle-bound, who stood over us counting "one-two-three," and kicking us or giving us a good thump when we made a mistake!

Most of us are intelligent enough to know that we need exercise; we are aware when our bodies get sluggish and do not respond to our commands as well as they should. But we dread the agony, exertion, and pain that we think we have to go through to become fit, and we put off doing something about it. Instead we make up a whole set of excuses: "I don't have enough time" or "In my kind of work I do not really need any exercise" or "I'm so exhausted at the end of the day, I figure I must have gotten some exercise in somewhere." These excuses are not worth the effort we put into making them up. Most of us know the truth, even though we do not admit it.

Some of us in the last few years have tried to do something about correcting our erring ways. We may have taken up jogging or signed up for an exercise class at the Y or a dance class somewhere. Usually these programs have confirmed our worst fears and dreads. We have strained our bodies beyond their limits, and the aches and pains have lasted for days afterward. And even after all that effort, there has not been a great change in the way we look or the way we feel.

Even worse has been what these programs can do to our pride. Many of us go into them feeling that we have to compete with each other or even with the instructors. We are made to feel — or even told outright — that we have to do these exercises as well as, or better than, the next person. If we can't, we are total failures. As a result we feel frustrated and demoralized. It rarely occurs to us that the instructor is a ''professional'' athlete, and his physical needs are much greater than ours. His body needs exercises that are severe because he has to have the strength and endurance for almost constant physical activity.

Most of us do not spend a large part of our time in athletic competition or hard physical labor, but our bodies nonetheless need a certain amount of exercise. This exercise can be pleasant and enjoyable, and it doesn't have to take more than 10 to 14 minutes each day. In fact, some exercises can be performed while going about ordinary routine tasks.

Before going into these exercises, however, it is important to change your attitudes about exercise in general, to get rid of the fear and dread, to realize that exercising is something you do *for* yourself, to make yourself feel better, not worse. You want to be able to climb a flight of stairs, or carry a heavy package, or run for a bus, without losing your breath or feeling dizzy. You exercise so that you will feel physically fit and can enjoy your life to the fullest.

You must also realise that you do not have to compete with someone else in the exercises you do. If you are competing with anyone, it is with yourself, with your own inertia. Get reacquainted with your body through seeing what you can or cannot accomplish. Let your body, your intake of food, and your daily activities be the determining factors.

And remember that you don't have to do all the exercises at the very beginning. Certainly do not attempt to do the most difficult and strenuous exercises the first few days. Start with the simplest and most basic, and build your regimen by gradually working in some of those that you know your body will resist. If you try an exercise and it proves to be extremely painful, do not force it; wait and try it after your body has become fully accustomed to those exercises you are already capable of performing. Of course, you should be aware that the more you are able to do, the more strength and endurance your body will have, and the more alert and alive you will feel.

Stand Up for Your Health

In getting to know your body better, take a look at the way you stand. You may not think it matters much, but it does. If you stand on your heels, for instance, your shoulders will tend to sag and sway back, you will place a strain on your sacroiliac, and your middle will go to paunch. Innumerable physical problems can result, problems that eventually might send you to a doctor in search of a remedy. It is much simpler, and less costly, to learn to avoid these problems before it is too late.

To stand correctly, get your weight off the heels. Center your weight over the feet, applying slight pressure to the inner ball of each foot. (To locate the balls of your feet, raise your toes. The spot where you feel pressure on each foot is the area that should share weight with the heels.)

Tighten you buttocks and tuck your pelvis under. This will put the organs of the pelvic area in their proper place, on the pelvic floor rather than leaning against the weak abdominal wall, which will give you a pot-bellied look. This also straightens the low part of your back, giving your spine a firm and level foundation.

Do not loosen your buttocks now. Anytime you are standing, your buttock muscles should be slightly contracted.

Now you are going to bring your upper torso into alignment. Do not anticipate a command of "shoulders back, chin up." That has been one of the most misunderstood rules of good posture. It is not precisely "shoulders back." We are going to concentrate on your shoulder blades. Using the muscles of your upper back (not your shoulders or your arms), pull your shoulder blades down and in toward your spinal column. As your shoulder blades squeeze toward the middle of your back, you will bring both your shoulders and your breastbone into correct position.

It is not precisely "chin-up" either. Concentrate on your neck; stretch your neck upward in line with the top of your head; the chin will follow into the correct position.

Your head should now rest perfectly on your spine. Your arms should be hanging loosely and comfortably alongside the body with the elbows straight and the palms of the hands turned toward your legs. If you haven't made a mistake somewhere along the line, your stance should be erect with a slightly forward lean. If your back is swaying, if you feel like you are going to fall over backward, read over the instructions again.

Breathe

Another thing most people do not know how to do is breathe. What? You say you have been doing it for years? Well, maybe so, but maybe not properly. If you are doing it the wrong way, you may be creating problems that will eventually land you in the doctor's office. A great many poor breathers deprive their muscles and brain of oxygen necessary to maintain good metabolism.

The most common error men make in breathing is to contract the diaphragm and expand the lungs, forcing the abdominal wall forward. Since the abdominal wall is not tightened with each exhalation, this soon creates a pot belly.

The most common mistake women make in breathing is to inhale by raising or lifting the rib cage. They think this will prevent a protruding belly. Instead it ventilates only the top of the lungs and creates too much tension in the muscles of the shoulders, neck, and throat, and causes the rib cage to grow rigid.

When you breathe correctly, your ribs spread with every breath, and your abdominal wall contracts every time you exhale. To learn to breathe correctly, try the following exercise:

Cup your hands over the lower ribs so that your fingertips meet. Inhale slowly as if you were smelling a flower; and, as you inhale, gently press your hands against the lower ribs, directing the ribs apart and to the sides, like an accordion. As you inhale, count to eight or ten. As you exhale, also to the count of eight or ten, open your mouth and breathe out with an audible sound like a sigh. As you exhale, you should feel your abdominal muscles tighten.

Now that you have learned to breathe, keep breathing.

Where to Find 14 Minutes a Day

If you have not been getting the proper exercise, very likely it is because you have been too busy, or at least you think you have been too busy. However, there are ways of finding the time to get your minimum daily requirement of exercise. If you cannot set aside a specific time of day when you concentrate on nothing else, you can at least incorporate exercise into some of your routine daily chores. Whoever you are, however you spend your day, there are ways of sneaking in some exercise — as you get out of bed in the morning, as you shower, shave or apply your make-up, move about the kitchen, go to the office, or even while you are working in your office. Always try to exercise in a warm — but not hot — room. Muscles work better and more easily when warm.

These exercises are intended to tone and firm your muscles so that they will respond properly when you need them. They are to be considered a minimum. You *should* get more exercise than this. However, if all you want is to get by with a minimum of time and effort, or if there are days when you cannot manage to set aside your 14 minutes, try these:

Waking Up

STRETCH

In the morning when you wake up, before you get out of bed, simply stretch. Stretch to your full ability and yawn as wide as you can. This is what a cat or a dog does after it has been sleeping, and it ought to come naturally to you, too. Stretch and enjoy it, with your arms, your legs, your entire body.

PRESS

Still in bed, bring each of your knees, one at a time, up to your chest, guiding them with your clasped hands. Keep the other leg flat out in front of you. First with one leg and then with the other, try to pull the knee down to touch the chest. (If you can't touch your chest, don't force it; just bring the knee down as far as you can.) Then straighten the leg. Do this about ten times with each leg.

If you don't have a weak back, you can follow this step with one in which you flatten your back to the bed and attempt to bring both knees up to your chest at the same time; but if you do have back problems, do not attempt it.

SIT-UP

This part of the exercise can be performed either on the bed or on the floor. (If you choose the floor, do the Toe Touch *before* you do the sit-up.) With your back flat on the bed or floor, bend your knees and draw your feet in so that the soles rest flat on the surface, close to your buttocks. Clasp you hands lightly behind your head and raise you torso off the bed, attempting to touch your knees with your elbows. As you do this, gently tighten your abdominal muscles. Do not strain, but try to get your elbows as close to your knees as you can. In the beginning, repeat this about five times; but in the following weeks or months, try to increase it to ten or fifteen times.

You can give this exercise a little twist, alternating touching your left knee with your right elbow; and your right knee with your left elbow. Remember, keep your abdominal muscles as tight as you can.

TOE TOUCH

It is now time to get out of bed. After you swing your feet over onto the floor, do not get up immediately. Sit on the edge of the bed and bend over and touch your toes four or five times. Then stand up and stretch as high as you can, as if you were trying to touch the ceiling. Continue to stretch for a count of ten to twenty.

JOG IN PLACE

On your way into the bathroom for your morning toilet, pause to run in place for a count of about 100 steps. As you improve, you can gradually build this to 200. Raise your knees as high as you can without pain. Do not worry if you get slightly out of breath. The object of this exercise is to get your pulse rate up to 120. (As I have indicated earlier, everyone should get the pulse rate up to 120 at least once a day, in order to put a load on the cardiovascular system.)

Bathroom Exercises

SCRUB

Time to take your shower or bath. As you are washing, rub your skin briskly with the washcloth; and as you are drying rub your body thoroughly and briskly with a large towel, especially over your back and legs. Part of the benefit of this is, of course, the exercise, but it will also help your circulation, particularly in bringing the supply of blood to the skin.

KNEE BEND

Now to the wash basin to brush your teeth. As you reach the basin, take hold of the edges and do ten to fifteen knee bends, going as far as you are able without causing pain. You can start with a half or three-quarters bend, and then gradually deepen it as your legs become more accustomed to the exercise. Eventually, you may be able to increase the number of knee bends to twenty or even thirty.

TOE-UP

As you brush your teeth and go about the remainder of your toilet, you can exercise your calves and ankles by rising up and down on your toes. You should be able to do anywhere between 45 to 75 of these. As you perform this exercise, try to remember to keep your abdominal muscles tight.

BUMPS

As you shave or put on your make-up, tighten your abdominal muscles and roll your pelvis forward, making sure to keep your gluteus maximus (or buttock) muscles tensed. Hold for counts of anywhere from 25 to 50; then relax and do it again.

LEG LIFT

When your morning toilet is completed, hold on to the wahbasin again and do six or eight leg lifts and twists. Do this first with one leg, then with the other, pointing your toes inward for a few lifts, then straight forward, and then slightly outward. You do not have to lift the leg extremely high to obtain benefits; just lift it as high as you can comfortably. Eventually you may want to increase this to ten or fifteen lifts with each leg. If you have a back problem, it is not advisable to kick your legs backward. Whether your back is weak or not, remember to keep it flat and not arched.

STRETCH

Now you can stand up and stretch, reaching as high as you can. Then clasp your hands behind your head and twist your neck — four times to the right, four time to the left — and roll your head around in a circular motion, first one way, then the other.

You should now feel considerably more refreshed and energetic than you would if you had sat down for a cup of coffee and a sweet roll.

Tub Exercises

You may look upon your bathtub as a special place where you like to relax, but exercise and relaxation go hand in hand; each is dependent upon the other. So you may find your bath is even more enjoyable if you spend part of your time there exercising. (Of course, it is very important to have a rubber mat or some of those nonslip decals in the tub to prevent an accident.) You can do your tub exercises in the evening when you have more time and feel less rushed.

To prepare for your bath exercises, fill the tub to drain level with warm water. When the tub is full, step in and slowly slip into the water. At first, lie back in the tub and relax, perhaps placing an inflatable plastic pillow under your head and a towel under your body.

RELAX YOUR LEGS

Lying back in the tub, let your legs float in the water for a few minutes.

STRETCH YOUR THIGHS

Lying back in the tub, with your knees bent, lift your feet out of the water, bring the soles together, and hold for a count of five. Then slowly bring your knees together, hold for a count of five, and relax by returning your feet to the water. Repeat five to ten times.

STRETCH YOUR LEGS

Sitting up in the tub, with your legs straight, flex your feet and reach out with your hands to grasp your ankles or your toes. First pull your right foot up so that your heel is out of the water; then lower it, and pull your left foot up. Repeat five to ten times. This is an excellent exercise for the legs and thighs.

SIDE PRESS

Sitting up in the tub, with your legs straight in front of you, spread your legs so that your feet touch the sides of the tub. Press your feet against the sides, and hold for a count of five; then relax and repeat eight to ten times. This will help to tone and firm the outer thighs.

LEG LIFT

Turn onto your right side, propping yourself on your right elbow. Prop your left leg up somewhere — perhaps against the faucet or the end of the tub — so that it is straight. Raise and lower your right leg out of the water to touch your left foot, keeping your legs straight and your abdomen tight. Repeat eight to ten times, then turn to your left side and repeat with your left leg. This will benefit the inner thighs.

KNEE SQUEEZE

Sit up in the tub with your knees up and your feet flat on the bottom of the tub. Place a washcloth between your knees, and squeeze it using only your knees, holding for a count of five. Then relax, wet the cloth, and repeat eight to ten times. This helps to firm the inner thighs.

LEAN-BACK

Sit up in the middle of the tub with your hands on your hips, your knees up in front of you, and your feet flat on the bottom of the tub. With your abdomen tight, lean back slowly as far as you can, then slowly return to your sitting position. This is rather difficult, and you should not expect to go all the way down; just try to keep your balance while you lean back as far as you can comfortably. (You should not do this if you have a weak back.) This exercise benefits the abdominal muscles. Repeat no more than five times in the beginning, and gradually increase the number over a period of weeks or months.

SHOULDER LIFT

Lie back in the tub with your legs stretched out as far as possible, and with your hands tucked under the small of the back, palms down. Tighten your stomach muscles, lift your head, and pull your shoulders forward as far as you can without straining. You should allow your elbows to bend out and forward as you lift. Hold for a count of ten, and return to starting position. Relax, then repeat five times in the beginning, increasing the number over a period of weeks or months. This benefits both your abdomen and your shoulders.

KNEE TOUCH

Lying back in the tub with your knees up and your feet flat on the bottom of the tub and your hands resting comfortably on your thighs, and keeping your abdomen tight, raise your right shoulder out of the water, lifting your right hand across to touch your left knee. Relax, and reverse the procedure, touching your left hand across to your right knee. Repeat eight to ten times. This benefits your abdomen, waist, and shoulders.

HIP LIFT

Sit up in the tub with your elbows bent behind you and with the palms of your hands braced against the rim of the tub. Make sure your hands are dry so that your grip is not slippery. Lift your hips out of the water, then lower them. Repeat five times in the beginning, increasing the number over a period of weeks or months. This is good for firming your upper arms and upper back.

ANKLE ROTATION

Either sitting or lying in the tub, lift your right leg and slowly rotate your right foot at the ankle in a clockwise direction five times; then reverse to a counterclockwise direction for the same number of rotations. Lower your leg, relax, and then repeat the exercise with your left foot. This exercise helps to strengthen the ankles.

FOOT FLEX

Lying back in the tub with your legs extended in front of you, lift your right leg, bending the knee, so that the toes point toward the bottom of the tub. Flex your foot and straighten out the leg so that the toes point back toward your head. Relax and repeat five times. Then repeat the exercise with your left leg and foot. This helps to stretch and tone your calves as well as to strengthen your ankles.

NECK ROTATION

Sitting up in the tub with your legs and arms relaxed, rotate your head in a slow clockwise motion eight to ten times. Then reverse to a counterclockwise motion for the same number of rotations. Don't worry if your neck pops and cracks. Nod back and forth a few times, then nod side to side. Relax. This helps to stretch and loosen your neck and shoulders.

Shower Exercises

I have already mentioned in the bathroom exercises that you should scrub your skin in the shower to wake up the circulation; but there are also exercises that you can perform in the shower *if you are very careful.* You must have a rubber mat or nonslip decals on the bottom, and you must have a secure shower rod or secure walls to brace yourself against. Do *not* do these exercises if there is the slightest possibility that the floor or sides of the shower are slick or soapy. You know your shower, so you be the judge, but be careful.

STRETCH

Standing on the balls of your feet, flex your toes, and stretch first one arm high overhead, then the other. Use the arm you are not stretching to brace yourself.

SHOULDER ROTATION

With your arms down at your sides, lift and rotate your right shoulder forward five times; then reverse and rotate the same shoulder back five times. Relax, and repeat the exercise with your left shoulder. This benefits the muscles of the shoulder and upper back.

SIDE STRETCH

Raise your right arm over your head, stretching it over to your left side. Stretch five times, then relax. Repeat with the left arm. If you keep your stomach in tight, this will help to trim the waist and firm the thighs.

BODY TWIST

Spread your legs apart, securing your feet against the sides of the shower if possible, keeping your stomach tight. Bend your elbows, and twist your torso back to the right so that your right elbow reaches behind your back. Then twist to the left. Repeat six or eight times. This benefits the shoulders, waist, and abdomen.

LEG TWIST

Do this exercise only if you can brace yourself against the shower walls. Stand in the center of the shower where your arms can extend out to the walls for support. With your stomach in tight, lift your right leg back so that your right heel stretches back behind your left leg. Return to the original position, shift your weight to your right leg, and repeat the exercise in reverse using your left leg and heel. Repeat six or eight times. This helps the waist, abdomen, and buttocks.

KNEE TWIST

Again, do not perform this exercise unless you can brace yourself securely against the shower walls with your hands. Holding on this way, raise your right leg, bending the knee, and secure the right foot behind the left thigh. Tuck in your stomach and twist, swinging your right knee left to right. Repeat six to eight times; then shift your weight to your right leg, and repeat the exercise with your left leg. This benefits the waist, thighs, abdomen, and buttocks.

KNEE LIFT

Hold on to the shower bar, or whatever you have that is secure. Take a deep breath and relax. Bring your right knee up toward your chest, as high as you can, then shift your weight to your right leg and lift your left knee. Repeat six to eight times. This benefits the abdomen and helps to straighten the knees.

Kitchen Sink Exercises

By this time you may feel you had everything but the kitchen sink thrust at you. Now you are going to get that as well.

If you spend a great deal of time in the kitchen, you might find it enjoyable to pause in your work from time to time and do a bit of exercise. You can easily use your sink or countertop in the way dancers use the ballet bar during practice; but do be careful dancing around the kitchen. (Make sure all pots and pans are out of your way.)

Like a dancer's bar, your kitchen sink or countertop will permit you to brace yourself with your hands so that you can exercise your legs, hips, and thighs with greater flexibility.

CALVES

Stand at a comfortable distance away from the sink, facing it, and gripping the edge with both hands. Stand erect, so that your head is up and your abdomen tucked in. Place your weight on your right foot, and lift yourself up and down on the toes of your right foot ten to fifteen times. Then shift your weight to the left foot and repeat the exercise.

ANKLES AND ARCHES

Continuing to stand facing the sink, with both hands holding on, place your weight on your right foot. Lift your left foot and place it behind your right ankle. Raise yourself up and down on the toes of the right foot ten to fifteen times. Then shift your weight to the left foot and repeat the exercise.

BUTTOCKS

Step away from the sink to arm's length, but continue to face the sink; holding on with both hands. Keep your abdomen tight and bend forward from the hips. Bend down as far as you can; if possible, get your head down below the top of the counter or sink. Keep both legs straight, but place your weight on your left leg, and raise and lower your right leg, pointing your toes. You may not be able to lift the leg more than a few inches off the floor, so do not force it. Raise and lower it eight to ten times while keeping your head down and your back straight from the hips. Then shift your weight to your right leg, and raise and lower your left leg eight to ten times.

HIPS AND WAIST

Stand away from the sink at arm's length, facing the sink and holding on with both hands. Place your weight on your left leg, and bring your right knee up as high as you can without straining. Swing your knee over across to the left, then back out to the right. Swing it left to right ten to fifteen times; then shift your weight to your right leg, and repeat the exercise with your left leg.

THIGHS 1

For this exercise, you must be able to get a good grip on the sink so that you do not fall. Standing facing the sink as far away as you can and still hold on with both hands. Lean back, balancing your weight on your toes, and bend your knees, coming down as far as you can. Then use your thighs to lift yourself up and down eight to ten times.

THIGHS 2

Stand with your left side to the sink or counter, holding on with your left hand. Standing erect, with your stomach in, place your weight on your left leg and raise your right leg as high as you can, bending the knee as it lifts. Then place your right hand under the right thigh for support, and straighten the right leg out in front of you. Bend and straighten the right leg eight to ten times; then turn your right side to the sink or counter, and repeat the exercise with your left leg.

INNER THIGHS 1

This is another exercise that requires a good grip on the sink. Stand facing the sink with your legs apart, at approximately shoulder width, and with both hands gripping the sink. You are going to shift between a knee bend to the right on your right leg and a knee bend to the left on your left leg. (As you bend down on one leg, the opposite leg will lift off the floor.) Bend down on your right leg, bounce twice, then come up; bend down on your left leg, bounce twice, and come up again. Repeat five to ten times.

INNER THIGHS 2

Stand facing the sink with your feet apart at approximately shoulder width, toes straight ahead. With your weight balanced on both feet, rise up on your toes, bend your knees, and lower your body as if you were sitting in a chair, keeping your abdomen in and your back straight and perpendicular. When you are down, "in the chair," hold for a count of five, then rise. Repeat eight to ten times.

WAIST

Stand with your left side to the sink or counter, holding on with your left hand. Raise your right arm straight up toward the ceiling, tuck in your abdomen, and bend over to touch your toes twice. Then straighten up, with your arm still extended over your head, and stretch it over your head to the left twice, bending your upper torso slightly to the left as you do. Then straighten up and repeat the exercise eight to ten times. Now turn your right side to the sink or counter and perform the exercise with your left arm.

HIPS

Stand with your left side to the sink or counter, holding on with your left hand. With your weight on your left leg, end your right knee and cross your right leg over in front of your left. As you do this, cross your right arm over your abdomen. Flex your right foot and swing both your right leg and your right arm out and back to previous position. Repeat eight to ten times; then turn your right side to the sink or counter, and repeat the exercise with your left leg and left arm.

Office Workers' Extras

Men and women who work in offices generally spend a large part of their day sitting. Most commute to work by automobile, park in a basement garage or lot on the premises, take an elevator, and hardly move from their offices until they have to repeat the procedure in reverse. Of course, if you work in an office, you do not need a great many extreme exercises, but you do need enough exercise to keep fit. There are a few simple extra movements you can do to get that extra bit of bounce and agility you need to keep on your toes.

THE THREE-BLOCK WALK

Instead of parking your car in the garage or just outside your office door, leave it a few blocks away from your office and walk the rest of the way. Even if it is only three blocks, the little bit of exercise you get from a short, brisk walk will benefit you. Besides helping your circulation, it may save you some money.

TAKE THE STAIRS

Do not depend so much on the elevator. If you are twenty or thirty floors up, of course you have to use the elevator — but only part of the way. Get off a few stops below your floor and walk up the rest of the way. In the beginning, you should try only two or three flights, but you can add a flight every few days or every few weeks, depending on how your cardiovascular system adjusts. (When you can climb three flights of stairs without getting out of breath, you know it is time to add another flight.)

Do the same thing when you leave the office. Walk down two or three flights, and then take the elevator the rest of the way. This will burn up a few calories, help the muscles of your legs, and limber up the joints of knees and hips.

DON'T SIT WHEN YOU CAN STAND

An executive does not always have to sit at his or her desk. There are times when you can stand — when someone comes in to confer briefly, when you have to read something, when you talk on the telephone. It may be convenient to ask your secretary to come to your desk; but if you occasionally walk over to his or her desk, *you* will get the benefits of that exercise. Also, if you have to speak to the person in the next office, don't use the phone; walk over. When you go to the restroom, try going to the one on the floor above or below your office — and go by the stairs!

The Exercise Break

Instead of having coffee in the middle of the morning or in the afternoon, try an exercise break. It is just as refreshing, and has more long-range benefits. There are a number of movements you can do in your office that will not make you appear foolish.

WALL PUSH-UP

Stand about two feet away from the wall, place your hands on the wall for support, and then lean. Push yourself back and forth from the wall ten or fifteen times. This will help the muscles of your shoulders and upper arms. As you adjust to this exercise, you can increase the number of times you do it. You can add further benefits by placing your hands so that the fingers of each hand point in toward each other. Or you can stand a little further back from the wall, so that you add more weight onto your arms.

DESK PUSH-UP

A variation of the wall push-up can be done at your desk. Standing a few feet away from the desk, rest your hands on the edge and do your push-ups.

LEG PRESS

An excellent exercise you can do seated at your desk is to cross your legs and press them against each other. This can be done in two variations: with your legs crossed at the thighs, and with them crossed at the ankles or calves. With your right leg over your left leg, press downward with the right while pressing upward with the left. Then reverse the legs, pressing down with the left and up with the right. When they are crossed at the ankles or calves, the pressure can be directed forward and backward. This exercise is excellent for the thighs, buttocks, and abdomen.

BODY LIFT

Another exercise that can be done seated at your desk involves leaning forward slightly, with your feet lightly on the floor and your hands on the arms of the chair, and pushing up. The object is to lift yourself from the chair using your arms and shoulders. In the beginning, you may have to help yourself along by using your feet, but eventually you should be able to lift yourself entirely with your arms, eight, ten, or even twenty times. This exercise is not recommended for those who are extremely overweight; and women may not wish to do it, because it can build the arms and shoulders to an extent that clothing will no longer fit properly.

Chapter 10

EXERCISES FOR MEN

Because office life is sedentary, business people often assume that they do not need much exercise. Too many of them do not realize how wrong they are until they develop high blood pressure, heart disease, or a respiratory ailment. The problem is that they cannot *see* what is really happening to them; all they can see is that they are getting a little paunchy in the middle, and that they do not move as well as they used to. But the really serious problems caused by lack of exercise are taking place inside their bodies, in the heart, lungs, circulatory system, muscles, and other organs.

The exercises in Chapter 9 constitute what I consider to be the *minimum* everyone should do just to keep mobile and alert for a normal day. Certainly, most people *should* do more than that, but I realize that most people are not sufficiently motivated to devote a specific time each day to nothing but taking care of themselves.

If, however, you are determined to achieve your ideal weight and keep sufficiently fit to live a longer, healthier, and happier life, you can set aside 14 minutes a day to devote to your body's upkeep. It should be time that is set aside from your normal routine, a time in which you get yourself into unrestricting workout clothes (something loose and comfortable) and down onto the floor, with nobody watching you to make you feel self-conscious. (At La Costa, we supply our guests with warm-up suits for the exercises. If you do not have a warm-up suit, wear whatever you have that will not restrict your movement. Do not wear something that fits tightly in the middle or in the crotch; wear as little as possible.)

You can select your own exercises from those that follow, but you should try to select a variety so that you work on all parts of your body — abdomen, neck, arms, thighs, buttocks, back, legs, and so on. Do not do the same ones every day; try to vary your choices. Always begin with a couple of warm-up exercises just to loosen up and get your heart working.

Of course, you should always begin an exercise program slowly. Do not attempt too much in the beginning. If you have been idle for a long time, notice the limits set for ''beginners'' on each exercise. Start with the recommended number of repetitions, and then work your way up.

If your object is to lose weight, do as many repetitions of each exercise as rapidly as you can. The secret of exercising to lose weight is to elevate your pulse rate to place a load on your heart, and work the muscles. If you perform the exercises slowly, you are toning and firming your muscles. If you are overweight, save that exercise approach until you are down to your ideal weight to keep from building up your muscles at the heavier weight. In toning and firming, the rule of exercise is to keep it as slow as possible, and to learn to breathe properly. For that reason, many of the exercises will have instructions on when and how to breathe. Do read the exercises carefully before you begin.

Warm-up Exercises

ARM SWING

Starting Position: Stand erect, with legs slightly apart. Beginning with your hands hanging loosely at your sides, raise your arms outward to just above shoulder height.

Exercise: Swing your arms across each other in front of your body; then out horizontally, back, and out again. Do not allow your arms to be tense; swing them from the shoulders, and keep them loose.

Repetitions: Beginners, eight to ten times; advanced, ten to fiteen times. Then stop and relax.

Benefits: Loosens the muscles of arms, shoulders, and back.

SHOULDER ROTATION

Starting Position: Stand erect with your feet comfortably apart, and raise your arms straight out to your sides at shoulder level, with your palms downward.

Exercise: Rotate your arms so that your hands form circles of approximately 18 inches in diameter.

Repetitions: This can be repeated ten to fifteen times by either beginners or advanced.

Benefits: Loosens arms and shoulders.

Variations: Turn the palms upward and reverse the direction of the circles.

DEEP-BREATHER

Starting Position: Stand erect with your arms down and in front of you, so that your hands rest on the front of your thighs.

Exercise: As you raise your arms out straight in front of you and up over your head, take a deep breath. Pull in your stomach, rise up on your toes, and hold for a count of two. Then, as you lower your arms, exhale and return to flat feet.

Repetitions: In the beginning, perform only five times, but gradually work up to twenty over a period of weeks or months.

Benefits: Improves the vital capacity of the lungs.

BODY TWIST

Starting Position: Stand erect, with your legs slightly apart. Lift your arms out to the sides to just below shoulder height.

Exercise: Twisting at the waist, swing your arms around. As the right arm swings in front of you, the left arm will swing back; then the left in front, the right in back. Do not tense your arms, but allow them to swing loosely. Keep swinging back and forth.

Repetitions: Beginners, five to ten times; advanced, ten to fifteen times; then stop and relax.

Benefits: Loosens the muscles of the arms, shoulders, and waist.

YOGA REVERSE SPINE
(See illus.)

Starting Position: Get down on your hands and knees with your haunches resting back against your heels so that your arms are stretched out in front of you.

Exercise: Tuck your chin under and inhale; shifting your weight to your arms, lunge forward, bringing your head up and back as far as you can, and exhale.

Repetitions: In the beginning, do this only five times, but eventually work up to ten or fifteen.

Benefits: Tenses the muscles of the thighs.

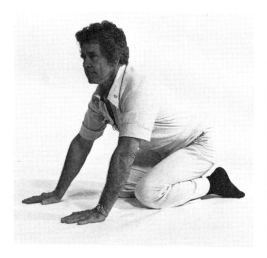

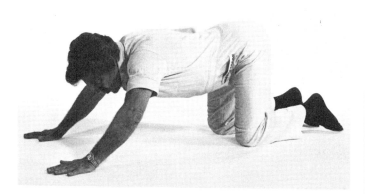

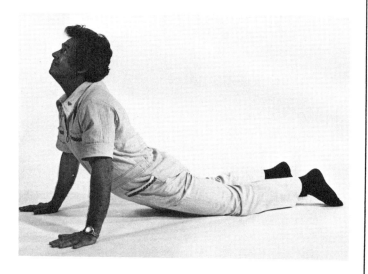

Yoga Reverse Spine

Neck, Back, and Shoulders

NECK and SHOULDER CURLS

Starting Position: Lie down flat on your back with your arms down at your sides.

Exercise: Raise your head up as far as you can, pull in your chin, and hold for a count of three. Keep the rest of your body flat on the floor. Then relax and return your head to the floor.

Repetitions: Beginners repeat five to ten times; advanced can increase to fifteen.

Benefits: Firms and strengthens the neck and abdominal muscles.

CHIN FIRMER
(See illus.)

Starting Position: Lie down with your back flat on the floor and spread your legs apart slightly.

Exercises: This exercise is done to the count of two. On the count of one, without lifting your back, lift your head and look at the heels of your feet. (This movement is the same as the Neck and Shoulder Curls.) On the count of two, again without raising your back, tilt your head back to look at the wall behind you.

Repetitions: Both beginners and advanced should repeat only four to five times; then relax. To relax your neck, sit up and roll your head around 360 degrees, first in one direction, then in the other.

Benefits: Strengthens the neck and firms the chin.

NECK STRETCH

Starting Position: Begin by lying down on your back and relaxing for a moment with your legs extended out flat on the floor, separated at about shoulder width.

Exercise: Pick a spot on the ceiling; raise your arm and point to that spot. Keep-

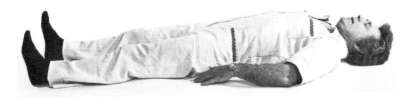

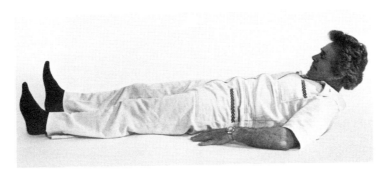

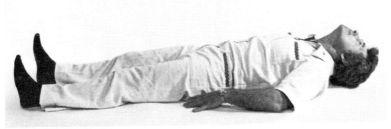

Chin Firmer

ing both eyes focused on the spot, and keeping your arm pointed up toward it, lift your head off the floor and try to touch your left ear to your left shoulder. Bring your head back to center, keeping it off the floor, then try to touch your right ear to your right shoulder. Bring your head back to center. Do this to the count of four — one, left; two, center; three, right; four, center — never letting your eyes slip away from the spot on the ceiling.

Repetitions: Both beginners and advanced should do this only four or five times; then relax. To relax your neck, sit up and roll your head around 360 degrees one way, then 360 degrees the other way.

Benefits: Strengthens and tones the neck muscles. It also benefits the muscles of the eye.

ARM STRETCH
(See illus.)

Starting Position: Get down on your hands and knees.

Exercise: Keeping your left hand on the floor, take your right hand and extend it, palm upward, through the space between your left hand and left knee. As you do this, follow your hand with your eyes, stretching that hand under as far as it will go three times. Then swing the arm back as far as possible, turning your head to follow the hand with your eyes. Stretch back as far as it will go three times.

Repetitions: Beginners, about five times with each hand; advanced, up to ten times with each hand.

Benefits: Helps to strengthen the muscles of the neck, shoulders, and back.

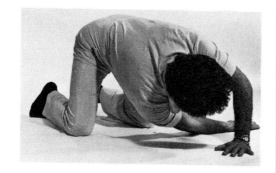

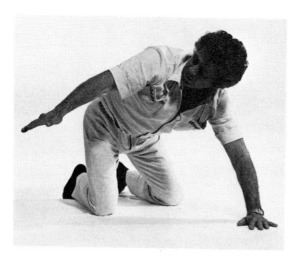

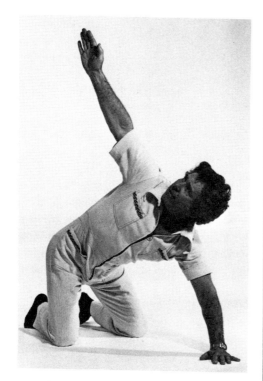

Arm Stretch

ROCK AND ROLL

Starting Position: Lie down on your back. Bring your knees up to your chest, and secure them there with your arms. Raise your head up so that you are resting on the small of your back and your tail bone.

Exercise: Rock back and forth — as far in each direction as possible while still retaining the proper position.

Repetitions: Beginners, five to ten times; advanced, ten to fifteen times.

Benefits: Tones the back and abdomen.

BACK-UP

Starting Position: Lie down with your back flat on the floor, with your legs bent so that your knees are up and your feet are flat on the floor as close to your buttocks as possible.

Exercise: Keeping your arms and shoulders down and your feet on the floor, lift your hips and lower back off the floor, raising them as high as you can and using your abdominal muscles to pull you up. Then, to lower yourself, gradually roll your back down, vertebra by vertebra, beginning with the upper back and ending with the hips.

Repetitions: Beginners repeat five times; advanced work up to ten.

Benefits: Helps to strengthen the legs, back, and abdomen.

Waist and Abdomen

KNEE RAISE

Starting Position: Lie down flat on your back with your legs straight and flat against the floor.

Exercise: Bring your head up and at the same time raise your right leg, bending the knee and bringing it toward your chest. Grasp the bent knee with both hands and pull it in toward your chest for a count of three. Pull in your abdomen and lower and straighten the leg; then perform the same exercise with your left leg.

Repetitions: Beginners, five times with each leg, alternating; advanced, ten times with each leg, alternating.

Benefits: Stretches the muscles of the leg and lower back and strengthens the muscles of back and abdomen.

SIDE LEG RAISE
(See illus.)

Starting Position: Lie down on your left side with your left arm extended. (If you are a beginner, you may prop your head on your elbow.) Allow your right arm to rest on the floor behind you as a brace.

Exercise: Raise your right leg straight up as far as you can, keeping the leg as straight as possible and keeping the abdomen tight. Raise the leg and lower it without allowing it to touch the right leg. Turn over to your right side to perform the same exercise with your left leg.

Repetitions: Beginners, five times each leg; advanced, ten times each leg.

Benefits: An excellent exercise for the leg muscles and hips and for trimming the "spare tire."

WAIST TRIMMER
(See illus.)

Starting Position: Lie down on the floor, knees bent and feet flat on the floor.

Exercise:

Step 1. Before doing the exercise, you are going to breathe. Start with your hands down at your sides, then slowly lift them upward over your head, taking a deep breath as you do. When they are directly over your head, tense them and stretch. As you exhale, allow your arms to relax and circle around to your side again.

Step 2. Place your hands behind your head, and — keeping your stomach muscles tight — lift your head up toward your knees. Do not pull yourself up with your hands and arms; your hands are behind your head simply to have a place to put them; and if you cannot reach your knees, do not

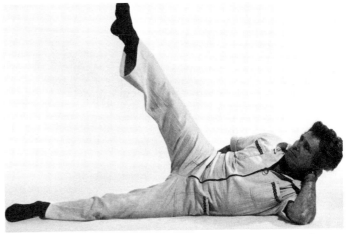

Side Leg Raise

force it. Simply roll upward, using your stomach and back.

Step 3. With your hands still behind your head and with your back flat, bring your knees up toward your head — up and down.

Repetitions: Beginners do each step three to five times; advanced, each step up to ten times.

Benefits: Trims and tones the waist, abdomen, and lower back.

Variations: After you have begun to get yourself into shape, you can extend this exercise by raising your head and your knees at the same time, up and down, trying to touch your elbows to your knees. This can be extended even further so that you twist when you lift, alternating between touching your left elbow to your right knee and your right elbow to your left knee.

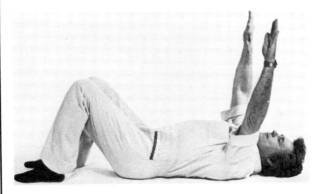

Waist Trimmer

(Waist Trimmer Cont.)

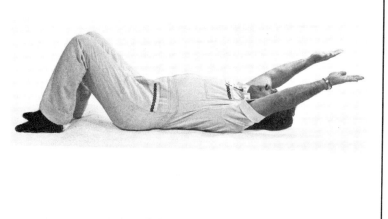

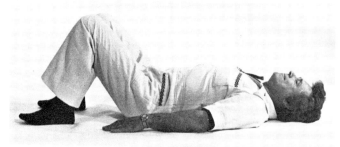

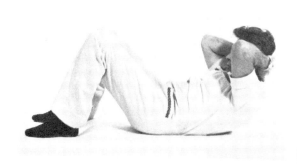

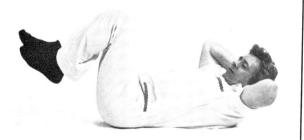

STRETCHING YOUR FLEXORS
(See illus.)

Starting Position: Lie down, with your back flat against the floor and your arms at your sides; then lift your legs up in the air, bending them to lift, but then straightening them so they are pointed toward the ceiling.

Exercise: Swing your legs around above you in a circular, clockwise motion for the repetitions you need. Stop, and swing them in a counterclockwise motion the same number of times.

Repetitions: Beginners, three to five rotations each direction; advanced, up to ten each direction.

Benefits: Tones and firms the hips, thighs, and waist. By performing this exercise as rapidly as possible for as long as you can stand it, you can use it for weight loss.

Variation: Try rotating each leg in the opposite direction, allowing one to cross over in front of the other. All the time you are doing this exercise, remember to keep the abdomen tight.

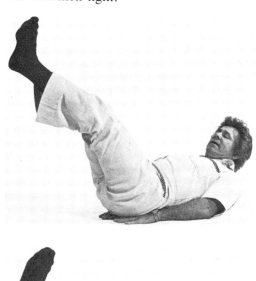

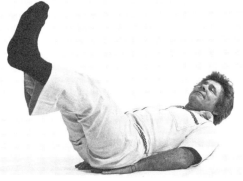

Stretching Your Flexors

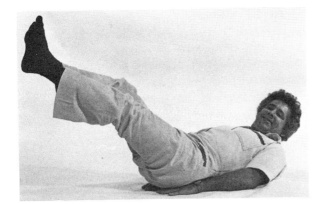

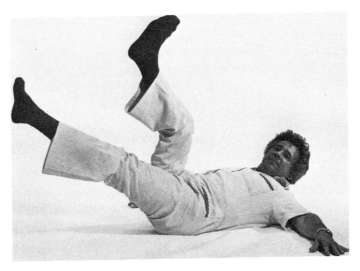

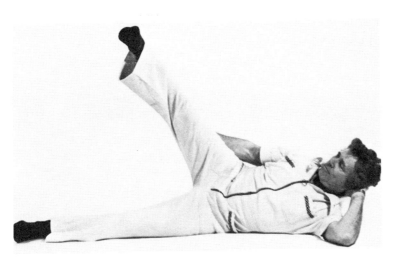

SIDE-TO-SIDE STRETCH

Starting Position: Stand erect with your feet apart at shoulder width.

Exercise: Keep your abdominal muscles tight as you lean to your left, bending the left knee and placing your weight on the left leg. As you do this, rest your left hand on your left knee and swing your right arm over your head, stretching it as far over as you can. Then shift your weight to your right leg and do the exercise to the right, with your right hand on your right knee and stretching your left arm over your head. Remember to keep your abdomen tight.

Repetitions: Beginners repeat five times each direction; advanced can gradually work up to twenty times each way over a period of weeks or months.

Benefits: Stretches all your side muscles and trims and firms the waist.

BODY TWIST

Starting Position: Stand erect with your feet apart at shoulder width; lift your arms, palms down, straight out from your sides at shoulder level.

Exercise: Keeping your abdomen tight, twist your body at the waist as far as you possibly can. Twist to the right, then to the left — back and forth, as far as you can go in each direction, allowing your arms to swing with each twist.

Repetitions: Beginners, five times each direction; advanced, ten to fifteen times each direction.

Benefits: An excellent exercise for toning and trimming the muscles of waist and hips.

BACK LEG RAISE 1

Starting Position: Lying down on your back, lift your torso up onto your elbows, with your hands resting under your hips.

Exercise: Slowly raise your left leg up as high as you can, trying to keep it straight, then return it to the floor. Follow by raising the right leg in the same manner.

Repetitions: Beginners repeat about five times with each leg; advanced can work up to fifteen or twenty with each leg over a period of weeks or months.

Benefits: Good for the muscles of the abdomen, legs, and lower back.

BACK LEG RAISE 2

Starting Position: Sitting on the floor, with your knees bent slightly and with your feet flat on the floor, place your hands on the floor out about a foot from your body and slightly back.

Exercise: Raise your hips and lower them.

Repetitions: Beginners repeat about five times; advanced can gradually work up to fifteen or twenty over a period of weeks or months.

Benefits: Helps to strengthen the muscles of the chest, shoulders, arms, and back. (If you keep your abdomen squeezed, it also helps to keep the midsection trim.)

Variation: Prop yourself back on your elbows rather than on your hands.

BACK LEG RAISE 3
(See illus.)

Starting Position: Get down on your hands and knees.

Exercise: With your head up, lower the lower portion of your back as much as you can; then raise it as high as you can, tucking your chin under, much the way a cat arches its back. Inhale as you lower; exhale as you arch.

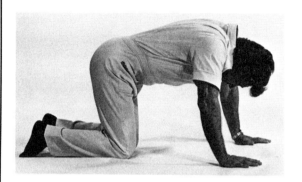

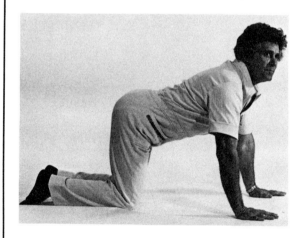

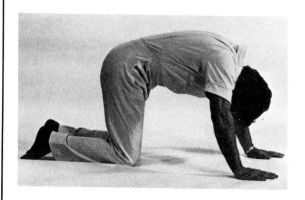

Back Leg Raise 3

Repetitions: Beginners can repeat this lowering and raising up to ten times; advanced can work up to as many as twenty times.

Benefits: Benefits the back and strengthens the muscles of the abdomen.

Variation: Support the upper torso on the elbows rather than the hands.

SIDE-SCISSORS
(See illus.)

Starting Position: Lie on your back and place your hands, palms downward, beneath your buttocks. Lift your legs straight into the air (bending your knees to lift, then straightening them), keeping your abdominal muscles tight.

Exercise:

<u>Step 1</u>. "Scissor" back and forth with your legs.

<u>Step 2</u>. Turn onto your left hip, propping your head with your left hand. Scissor out to the left.

<u>Step 3</u>. Shift onto your right hip and scissor out to the right.

Repetitions: Beginners, scissor back and forth five to eight times each direction; advanced, ten to fifteen times each direction.

Benefits: Helps to trim and firm the abdomen, hips, and thighs. If you wish to use this exercise for wieght loss (particularly steps 2 and 3), simply scissor as many times as you can, as rapidly as you can.

Legs, Thighs, Buttocks

THE BICYCLE

Starting Position: You are probably familiar with this one. But we won't make you lift yourself up onto your shoulders. Just lie down with your back flat against the floor and lift your legs up into the air, knees bent.

Exercise: Pedal the bicycle. Count as you go to keep yourself breathing properly.

Repetitions: Beginners or advanced,

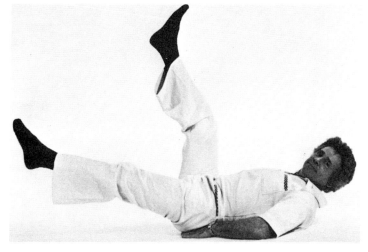
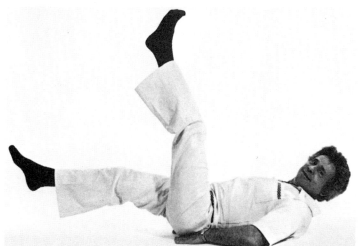
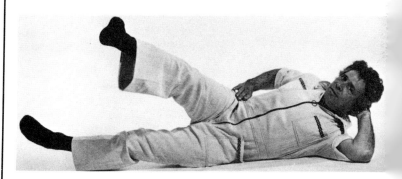
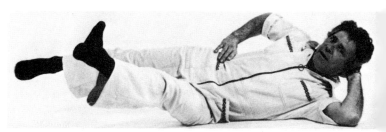

Side Scissors

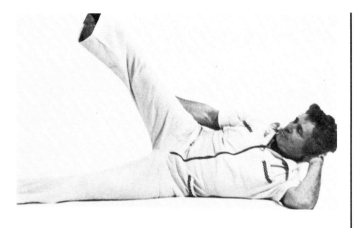

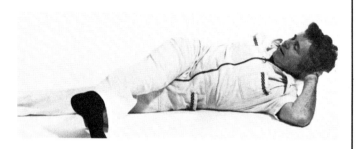

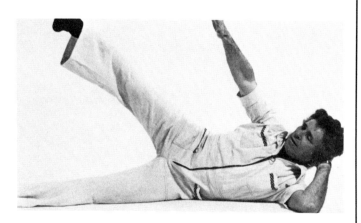

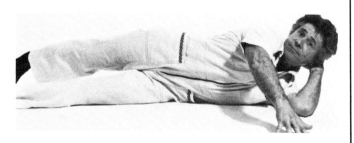

The Karate Blade

pedal as long as you can. (Beginners, probably ten times; advanced twenty.)

Benefits: Helps to trim and firm the thighs, hips, and waist. You can use this for weight loss by cycling as long and rapidly as possible.

THE KARATE BLADE
(See illus.)

Starting Position: Lie down on your left side, propping your head with your left hand. You are going to make a "karate blade" with your right foot. That means that you are going to turn your foot 90 degrees toward the floor. Extend that leg out in front of you, and extend your right arm out behind your back.

Exercise: Swing your right leg up high into the air and then down behind while swinging your right arm from behind to in front of you. Hand and foot should almost meet as they swing by each other directly over your body. Swing them up and over. Turn over onto your right side to repeat the exercise with your left leg and left arm.

Repetitions: Beginners, five to eight times each side; advanced, ten to fifteen times each side.

Benefits: Helps to firm and trim the buttocks, hips, and legs. This can be used for weight loss by performing the exercise as many times and as rapidly as possible.

THE JUDO SQUAT

Starting Position: Stand erect with your feet apart at shoulder width. Place your hands on your hips.

Exercise: Bend your knees to bring yourself down to a slight squat, keeping your back perfectly straight and vertical and your abdomen tight. Squat only about one-quarter of the way down, hold for a count of five, then raise yourself erect again.

Repetitions: Beginners, five to eight times; advanced, ten to fifteen times.

Benefits: Firms the leg muscles.

Variation: After you have accomplished this without difficulty, squat halfway down so that your thighs are parallel to the floor (with knees bent not more than 90 degrees). Hold for a count of five.

FRONT LEG RAISE

Starting Position: Lie down on your stomach, with your arms down at your sides, palms downward, and with your legs together.

Exercise:

<u>Step 1</u>. Raise your legs off the floor for a count of ten, then lower them.

<u>Step 2</u>. Separate your legs so that your feet are apart at about shoulder width. Place your hands palms downward under your chin and lock your fingers. Raise your head and shoulders off the floor for a count of ten; then relax.

<u>Step 3</u>. Bring your legs back together, keeping your hands clasped under your chin. Raise your head and shoulders and your legs simultaneously for a count of ten.

Benefits: This series helps strengthen the muscles of the back, legs, and buttocks.

Chapter 11

EXERCISES FOR WOMEN

Some of the exercises that we have prescribed for men can be performed by women as well. However, we do not recommend all of them because a woman's body is structured somewhat differently from a man's. For that reason, the women's program is also structured somewhat differently. If women did some of the exercises that we recommend for men (and vice versa), they might begin to overdevelop muscles in the "wrong" places, and their clothes would no longer fit properly.

The main distinction is that the women's exercises are not quite so strenuous and violent as the men's. But we also concentrate on different parts of the body. A man's fat generally accumulates around the middle, whereas the fatty places on a woman are most commonly the buttocks and the upper arms.

The women's exercises are gentler and more fluid than the men's, and they concentrate more on movement and flow and less on power and force.

To aid in that flow and movement, we recommend that you select a favorite piece of music to exercise by, preferably something lively and upbeat. Put a record or a stack of records on your phonograph, and you will find that your exercises will be easier and more enjoyable as your body responds to the rhythm.

Most women who are homemakers generally get more exercise in their daily activities than men do, but it is usually the wrong type of exercise. Although they are on their feet much of the day, very little of their work is strenuous, and very little of it exercises the important muscles. It is a relatively passive type of activity, moving at an unhurried pace from one place to another. They may very well feel exhausted at the end of the day, but it is generally not from having strained their muscles.

Actually, if they are to keep fit, women need heavier exercise than simple housework, because their bodies tend more toward fat than men's do.

The object of the exercise program for women is to tone and firm those parts of the body that get little exercise. It is not to build up muscles, but to prevent muscles from sagging and drooping, especially if you are intent upon losing weight.

These exercises are also excellent for getting a woman back into shape after childbirth. (A great many women spend a week or two at La Costa after a pregnancy, and many return after each birth, realizing how important the exercises are for maintaining good physical condition.)

Whether you are a homemaker or a businesswoman, you should find 14 minutes a day, at a regular time, when you do nothing but concentrate on exercises. It is important for your health and appearance and for the way you feel.

Before beginning your exercise program, read through the exercises offered and select from them. Don't do all of them every day, and don't concentrate on only one part of the body. Vary your daily program, but be sure to cover each area of the body at least twice a week.

It is also important to wear something comfortable and unrestricting, the less the better. A leotard, worn without a bra, is ideal for floor exercises. Certainly do not wear something you will worry about perspiring in.

If you haven't exercised for some time, start your exercise program slowly. Don't strain yourself too much too soon, because you might be tempted to give up at the first sign of aching muscles.

If you are trying to lose weight, do your exercises as quickly as possible so that you speed up the heart, burn up calories, and perspire. If you exercise slowly when you are overweight, you tend to firm up what you already have, so save that until after you have gotten down to your ideal size.

Warm-up Exercises

JOG AROUND

Starting Position: After putting your upbeat music on the phonograph, stand in the middle of the floor where you won't bump into anything.

Exercise: Jog in place in time to the music for a few moments. Remember to keep lifting your knees high. As soon as you have got the rhythm, jog around in a little circle to the right; then in a little circle to the left. Lift your knees high, and come down on your toes. Most people jog with their arms bent at the elbows, but if you are jogging to music, you can do anything you want to express yourself — swing your arms, reach for the sky, and so on.

Repetitions: About 20 to 50 steps in each direction.

Benefits: Gets the circulation going and loosens up your body. When you jog, increase your speed to lose weight, and decrease your speed to tone up the muscles.

THE GROUCHO WALK

Starting Position: Stand erect with your abdomen tight.

Exercise: Bend your legs and walk with the knees bent. Walk in a circle around to the right, and then around to the left. The more you can bend the knees, the better off you will be, but do not strain yourself. When you have finished, take a deep breath and exhale.

Repetitions: Walk until the muscles begin to ache.

Benefits: Helps to firm up the buttocks, and loosens the legs and abdomen.

CHICKEN WING
(See illus.)

Starting Position: Stand with your feet apart at shoulder width. Do a little bump to get your buttocks tucked under, and tighten and flatten your abdomen. Lift your arms out at the sides and bend them so that your elbows stick out parallel to the floor and your hands extend back toward your chin. (Your arms will look a little like chicken wings, and you will feel a slight pull at the waist and the lower back.)

Exercise: Keeping your arms out in this position and your abdomen tucked in, twist and bend your knees in time to the music. Twist your upper torso twice to the right, while you bend your knees, then twice to the left.

Repetitions: Beginners continue back and forth five to ten times; advanced, ten to fifteen times.

Benefits: Good for the waist and legs.

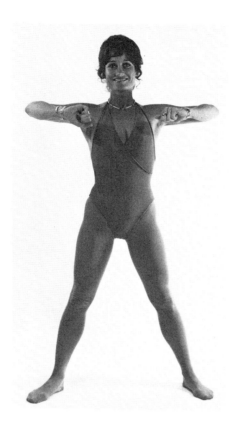

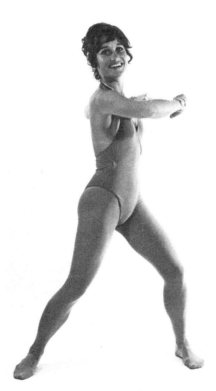

Chicken Wing

FLYING
(See illus.)

Starting Position: Stand with your feet apart at shoulder width, and bend slightly at the waist, keeping your abdomen tight.

Exercise: Remaining bent at the waist, swing your arms out and slightly back two times; then swing them back to cross in front of you two times.

Repetitions: Continue swinging arms back and forth ten to fifteen times.

Benefits: Loosens the arms, and helps firm up the fatty part of the upper arms, and trims and firms the fatty part of the back just behind the bra strap.

Waist and Abdomen

TOWEL EXERCISE 1

Starting Position: You will need a bath towel for this exercise. Stand erect, stomach in, feet apart at shoulder width. Roll the towel and grasp one end with your left hand, the other with your right.

Exercise: With your arms straight, and with the towel pulled taut, raise it high overhead. Remembering to keep the abdomen tight, bend twice to the right, twice to the left.

Repetitions: Beginners, five to eight times; advanced, eight to ten times.

Benefits: Helps trim and firm the waist.

CRISSCROSS 1

Starting Position: Lying flat on your back with your arms extended outward, raise both legs up toward the ceiling and spread them as far as you can without straining your back. (To keep from straining your back, bend your knees as you raise your legs; then straighten them up toward the ceiling.)

Exercise: Swing one leg across the other, and at the same time swing your arms up and across over your chest, lifting your head from the floor. As you swing your legs apart, swing your arms apart, and lower your head to the floor.

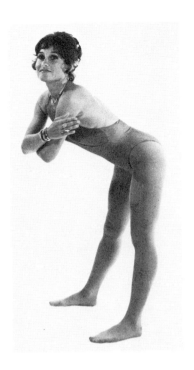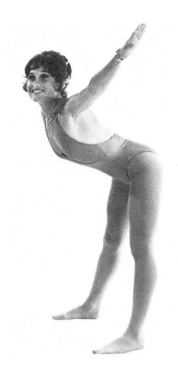

Since you are exercising a great many muscles at once, it is a good idea to count out loud to keep yourself breathing properly. Use a two count: one as you cross your legs and arms and lift your head, two as you part them.

Repetitions: Beginners, five to eight times; advanced can work up to ten to fifteen repeats.

Benefits: Excellent for the waist and abdomen, but also benefits the shoulders, thighs, and neck. You can use this exercise for weight loss by repeating as many times and as rapidly as you can.

SCISSOR VARIATIONS

Starting Position: Sit on the floor with your legs together straight out in front of you and lean back on your elbows. Bend your knees up to your chest, and then straighten them out above you, with toes pointed toward the ceiling. Your weight should be resting on your lower back, not on your tailbone. Your back should be comfortably rounded, not arched.

Exercise: With your legs up in the air, and with your abdomen tight, cross your

right leg over your left and back several times; then cross your left over your right and back several times. Then swing your left leg forward, and your right leg down almost to the floor; reverse the action in a scissor like motion with the right leg forward and the left down almost to the floor.

Repetitions: Beginners may be able to do three to five repeats of the first variation and three to five repeats of the second; advanced can repeat both variations five to ten times.

Benefits: Trims and firms the waist and abdomen, and tones up the lower back, buttocks, and thighs. You can use the scissor variations for weight loss by repeating them as many times and as rapidly as you can.

TOWEL EXERCISE 2

Starting Position: Stand erect, stomach in, feet apart at shoulder width. Roll a towel and grasp one end with your left hand, the other with your right.

Exercise: With the towel pulled taut, lift it high overhead. Then, keeping your abdomen tight, bend and twist to the right twice, then bend and twist to the left twice. (As you twist to the right, your right arm will swing behind you and your left in front; and as you twist to the left, your left arm will swing back and your right in front.)

Repetitions: Beginners, five to eight times; advanced, eight to ten times.

Benefits: Good for the waist, abdomen, and lower back.

SIT-UP
(See illus.)

Starting Position: Most people have a problem with sit-ups because they have been taught to do them the wrong way. There is no real benefit in having your legs straight and flat on the floor; and there is the possibility that you can do harm to your back by jerking yourself up. We recommend a modified sit-up that you can do even if you already have a weak back.

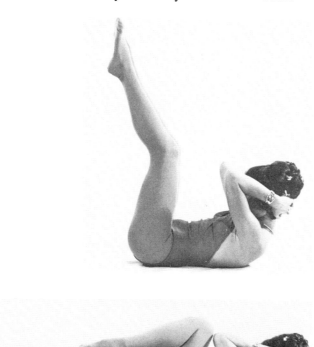

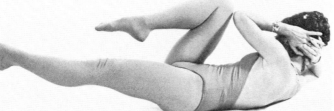

Sit-up

Lie down flat on your back on the floor. Place your hands behind your head, and pull in your abdomen. With your knees slightly bent, raise your legs almost striaght up in the air.

Exercise: You are going to attempt to touch your knees with your elbows. (If you cannot reach your knees in the beginning, do not worry, and do not strain.) As you perform these sit-ups, count out loud to keep yourself breathing properly. Sit up and exhale on the count of one, and lie back and exhale on the count of two.

Repetitions: Beginners, five or six times; advanced can work up to ten or fifteen times over a period of weeks or months.

Benefits: The object of the sit-ups is to firm up the muscles of the waist and abdomen, so remember to keep your stomach muscles in and tight, so you do not build them out into a pot belly instead of in. You can use the sit-ups for weight loss if you perform them rapidly.

Variation: By twisting with each sit-up and trying to touch the left elbow to the right knee (and vice versa), you can also benefit the legs, thighs, back, abdomen, and hips.

CHAIR-UPS

Starting Position: You will need a chair or stool for this. Lie down flat on your back with the lower part of your legs resting on the chair or stool.

Exercise: Place the palms of your hands loosely on your thighs, hold your stomach in tight, and raise up so your fingers slide along your thighs toward your knees. Reach as far up as you have to in order to feel a slight tightness in the abdomen.

Repetitions: Beginners, five to eight times; advanced, eight to ten times.

Benefits: Good for the waist and abdomen. You will also feel this in the back of the neck as you exercise, but that is normal. It is helping your neck muscles and chin, too.

SIDE BEND

Starting Position: Stand straight, with your feet together. Keep your stomach tucked in and your arms down at your sides.

Exercise: Bend from side to side, trying to touch each knee with your fingertips. Stretch three to four times toward each knee before switching to the other side. Do not bend forward at all; bend only to the side, and simply slide your hands down your thighs.

Repetitions: Beginners, four to eight times each side; advanced, eight to ten times each side.

Benefits: Tones and firms the waist and hips.

LEAN-BACK
(See illus.)

Starting Position: Sit on the floor with your knees flexed, and with your feet secured beneath a heavy armchair, bed, or sofa, with your back upright, and with your arms extended out toward your knees.

Exercise: Lean back approximately 45 degrees and hold for a count of ten to fifteen, keeping your abdomen tight. Then raise yourself back to the sitting position.

Repetitions: Three to five for beginners; five to ten for advanced.

Benefits: Ideal for the toning of the waist and abdominal muscles. This exercise can be done by those with a weak back who cannot normally do sit-ups. The lean-back substitutes very well for a complete sit-up.

Variation: After you have mastered the 45-degree angle, you can lower to a 60- or 70-degree angle.

Hips, Thighs, and Buttocks

HIP STRETCH
(See illus.)

Starting Position: Get down on your hands and knees.

Exercise: Lift your right leg up behind you, and stretch it across over your left foot. As you do this, stretch your neck to look over your left shoulder at your right foot. Shift your weight to your right knee, and repeat the exercise with your left leg over your right foot, stretching to look over your right shoulder.

Repetitions: Beginners, five to eight times each direction; advanced, eight to ten times each direction.

Benefits: Tones and firms the hips and thighs, and also aids the neck and back.

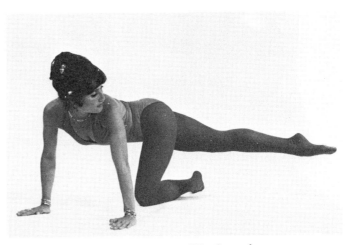

Hip Stretch

BODY ROLL
(See illus.)

Starting Position: Do not attempt this exercise if you have a weak back. Lie down on your right side with your right arm extended and with your left hand in front of you on the floor.

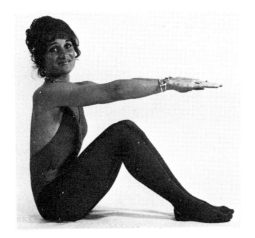

Lean-Back

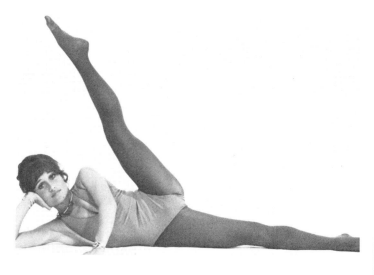

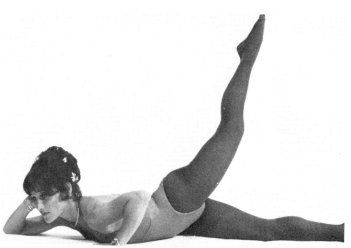

Body Roll

Exercise: Raise your left leg as high as you can, then roll over onto your stomach, keeping your leg in the air, but allowing it to turn with your body and causing your back to arch. Repeat. Then switch to your left side and repeat the exercise with your right leg in the air.

Repetitions: Beginners, five times each way; advanced, six to eight times each way.

Benefits: Tones and firms the hips and thighs.

HIP SWING

Starting Position: Lie down on your back, with your arms extended outward, palms down, and your legs lying flat and together.

Exercise: Keeping your abdomen tight and your knees together, bring your knees up over your stomach. Continuing with the knees tight together, swing them slowly over to the right until your right hipbone touches the floor. Bring them back over your stomach, then swing to the left until your left hipbone touches.

Repetitions: Beginners swing six to eight times each way; advanced, eight to ten.

Benefits: Excellent for the hips, thighs, abdomen, and waist. For weight loss, repeat as many times and as rapidly as you can.

CRISSCROSS 2
(See illus.)

Starting Position: Lie down on your stomach, with your hands clasped under your chin. (This is not recommended for those with weak backs.)

Exercise:

Step 1. Cross your left leg over your right and touch the floor; then cross your right over your left and touch the floor, keeping the knee straight.

Step 2. Raise your left leg up behind you as high as you can, then lower it and raise your right leg as high as you can.

Repetitions: Beginners can repeat six to eight times each leg, for each step; advanced, eight to ten times each leg, each step

Benefits: Helps to trim and firm the back of the thighs and the buttocks.

LEG SWING

Starting Position: Lie down flat on your back, with your arms stretched out to your sides. (Your arms will serve to brace you and keep your shoulders flat against the floor.)

Exercise: Raise your right leg straight up toward the ceiling, and swing it over

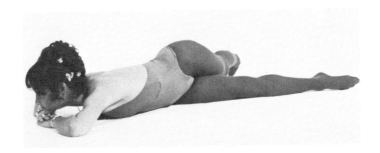

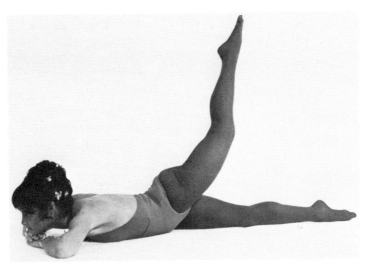

Crisscross 2

toward your left hand. Then swing the right leg over toward your right hand. Allow your hips to twist over, but keep your shoulders flat and your stomach tucked in. Repeat the exercise with your left leg.

Repetitions: Beginners, six to ten times each leg; advanced, ten to fifteen times each leg.

Benefits: Helps to trim and firm the muscles of the abdomen, hips, and thighs.

Variation: Bend both knees, and raise both legs up toward the ceiling, keeping them tight together. Swing both legs together in a clockwise circular motion. Then reverse the direction and form counterclockwise circles. Again, be sure to keep your stomach tight and your shoulders flat against the floor. Beginners can manage five to eight circles each way; advanced, eight to ten. This variation is not recommended for anyone with a weak back.

THIGH SLIMMER (FRONT)
(See illus.)

Starting Position: Sit on the floor, with your legs stretched out in front of you and your feet 8 to 10 inches apart. Lean back on your hands slightly (without bending your elbows) and tuck in your stomach. Flex your left foot. (Do not point your toes.) When the foot is flexed, your toes will be directed toward the ceiling, stretching the calf muscles.)

Exercise: With your left foot flexed and your left knee locked, raise your right leg up and down without touching the floor. You do not have to raise it more than 10 to 15 inches off the floor; height does not matter. The important thing is to keep your foot flexed and your knee locked. Repeat the exercise with your right leg.

Repetitions: Beginners, five to eight times each leg; advanced can work up to ten or fifteen over a period of weeks.

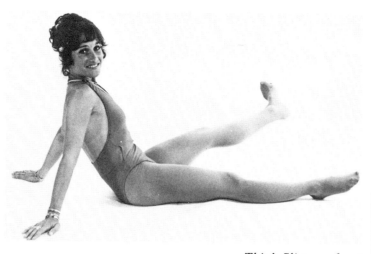

Thigh Slimmer-front

Benefits: Tones and trims the muscles on the front of the thigh.

THIGH SLIMMER (INNER THIGH)
(See illus.)

Starting Position: Sit on the floor with your legs out in front of you, spread in a comfortable position. Lean back and brace yourself with your hands resting on the floor.

Exercise: To work on the left thigh, flex your left foot, turning it out toward the left side. Shift your weight to your left hip, and lift the left leg up and down without touching the floor.

For the right leg, shift your weight to the right hip, flex your right foot, pointing it out toward the right, and raise and lower.

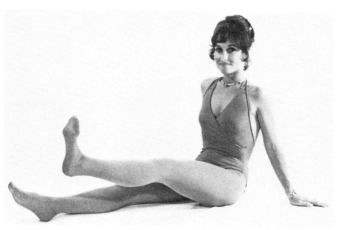

Thigh Slimmer—inner

Repetitions: Beginners may be able to repeat only five to eight times; advanced may be able to work up to ten or fifteen over a period of weeks.

Benefits: Tones, firms, and trims the muscles of the inner thigh.

Variations: As you improve with this exercise, finding yourself able to repeat fifteen to twenty times, you may want to add more weight to the lift. To do this, simply tuck the foot you are not using up toward your inner thigh.

You may also vary it by lying down on your back, legs straight up in the air, heels together and feet flexed outward. Spread your legs apart and back together. Beginners can manage five to eight repeats; advanced up to fifteen repeats.

THIGH SLIMMER (OUTER THIGH)
(See illus.)

Starting Position: To work on your left thigh, lie down on your right side, resting your torso on your left arm. Beginners will support themselves on the left elbow; advanced, on the left hand with elbow bent.

Exercise: Flex your left foot, turning it inward so that it is directed toward the floor, and raise and lower the left leg without allowing it to touch the floor. Keep the knee locked as you raise and lower the leg.

Turn over onto your left side, and repeat the exercise with your right leg.

Repetitions: Beginners raise and lower each leg six to eight times; advanced, eight to ten times each leg, or until you feel tired.

Benefits: Tones, firms, and trims the muscles of the outer thigh.

THIGH SLIMMER (BACK)
(See illus.)

Starting Position: Get down on your hands and knees.

Exercise: Keeping your stomach tucked in tight, extend your right leg out to the right so that you can see it, flex your

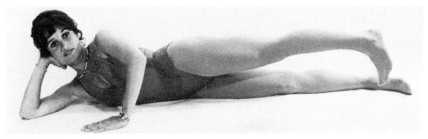

Thigh Slimmer—outer

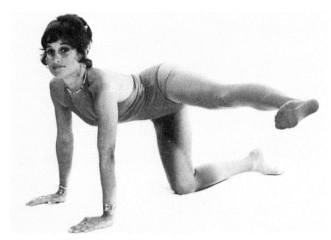

Thigh Slimmer—back

foot, and raise and lower your right leg without touching the floor. Keep your weight on your left knee as you raise and lower. Shift your weight to your right knee, and repeat with the left leg.

Repetitions: Beginners, six to eight times each leg; advanced, eight to ten times each leg, or until the muscle begins to ache.

Benefits: Trims and firms the back of the thigh and the buttocks.

Variation: You can vary this exercise to concentrate on your buttocks. Instead of lowering your leg, swing the leg up toward the shoulder and then return to the side, without putting it down. You may not be able to repeat this more than five times in the beginning, but you can increase it with time.

SKIER'S SQUAT
(See illus.)

Starting Position: Place your back against a wall, your feet far enough from the wall so that you can squat, with your calves perpendicular to the floor and your thighs parallel to the floor.

Exercise: Sit and hold this position until your thighs begin to ache; then rise up on your toes and push your body up to a standing position with your back still flat against the wall.

Repetitions: Beginners can repeat three to five times; advanced, five to ten times.

Benefits: Strengthens the thighs, legs, and feet.

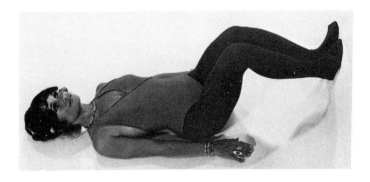

Skier's Squat

Bust, Back, and Arms

THE CAT

Starting Position: Get down on your hands and knees.

Exercise: Tuck your chin in, and round your back the way a cat does when it is angry. As you are lifting your back, exhale; as you lower your back and raise your head, inhale.

Repetitions: There is no limit to the number of times you can repeat this exercise. We recommend that you do it five to six times in the beginning and work up to ten to fifteen.

Benefits: Improves breathing and strengthens the muscles of the back.

HAND PRESS

Starting Position: Sit up straight, with your legs folded beneath you Indian-style. Place the heels of your hands together, fingers of each hand pointing in opposite directions, elbows pointing outward.

Exercise: Press your hands together, and release.

Repetitions: Repeat ten to fifteen times.

Benefits: Firms up the fatty part of the upper arm and helps firm the breasts. But be sure to keep your arms up and in, close to your chest; if you lower your elbows toward your body, the exercise will not be as effective.

Variations: You can vary this exercise by altering the position and direction of the hands. For example, you can place palms together, fingers pointing upward, or you can grasp and lock wrists.

PUSH-OFF
(See illus.)

Starting Position: Stand facing a wall, approximately two feet away. Extend your arms and lean against the wall with your hands directed in so that your fingers point

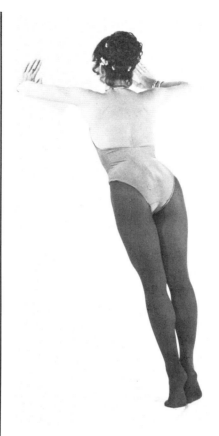

Push-off

toward each other. Roll up on the balls of your feet.

Exercise: Keeping your feet together and your abdomen tight, simply push yourself back and forth off the wall. If is too easy, move your feet further from the wall and increase your speed. If it is too difficult, move closer to the wall.

Repetitions: Beginners, five to eight times; advanced, eight to ten times.

Benefits: Good for firming the breasts and toning the arms and shoulders.

ARM-LEG WRESTLE
(See illus.)

Starting Position: You can work on your arms, bust, and legs at the same time with this exercise. Sit on the floor with your knees up in front of you, feet flat on the floor. Place your hands between your knees, palms outward.

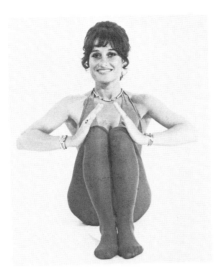

Exercise: As you press outward with your hands, trying to separate the knees, press in with your knees, trying to keep your hands together.

So that you exercise both sides of your arms and both sides of your thighs, reverse this exercise. Place your hands on the outside of your knees and press in, while you try to push outward with your knees.

Repetitions: Beginners repeat each variation five to eight times; advanced, repeat each eight to ten times.

Benefits: Tones and firms the muscles of arms, bust, and shoulders, as well as the muscles of the thighs.

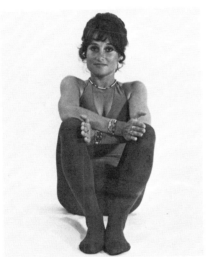

Arm-Leg Wrestle

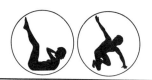

Chapter 12

COUPLE EXERCISES

The preceding exercise programs have been set up so that you can perform them alone, in the privacy of your home, without having someone looking over you to see how well you are doing them. I do not look upon exercise as a competitive sport; I feel it is something you owe your body.

If you enjoy the spirit of competition, however, and if exercising with someone will give you the incentive you need, go ahead, get together with your spouse or a friend, and have a good time. You can perform any or all of the individual exercises in company as well as alone; and there are some additional exercises you can do that require two people. They are excellent for strengthening, toning, and firming, and they are fun to do.

Arms, Shoulders, and Chest

WRIST WRESTLE
(See illus.)

Starting Position: You and your partner sit on the floor facing each other with your legs crossed Indian-style. (If you are unable to manage this position, cross your ankles, with your knees slightly up.) You should sit fairly close to each other, so that your wrists will cross when you extend your right arms with elbows slightly bent. Begin with the inside of your wrists meeting.

Exercise: You apply pressure to your left, while your partner applies pressure to his or her left, each of you trying to press the other's arm out of the way. Say "Go," apply pressure, count to five, and relax. Position the same wrists back to back. Each of you apply pressure to the right this time. Repeat the same number of times, then switch to the left wrists, and perform the exercise in both variations.

Repetitions: Repeat five or six times each way.

Benefits: Helps to strengthen and firm the muscles of the arms. If you play tennis, it will give you considerably more power for your forehand and backhand.

BACK WRESTLE
(See illus.)

Starting Position: Be careful not to strain yourself on this one if you happen to be a bit weaker than your partner. Sit back-

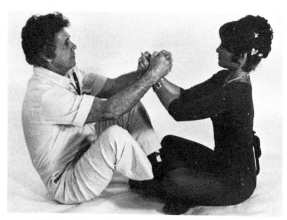

Wrist Wrestle

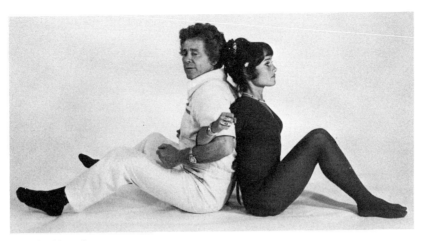

Back Wrestle

to-back, with your knees up and your feet flat on the floor.

Exercise: Lock arms with your partner, and pull back and forth for a count of five.

Repetitons: Relax, and repeat six to eight times.

Benefits: Good for the shoulders and arms.

TOWEL TUG 1
(See illus.)

Starting Position: You will need two bath towels for this and the next two exercises. You and your partner sit on the floor facing each other with your legs spread and knees locked tight; the soles of your feet are flat against the soles of your partner's feet.

Have the two towels stretched out taut between you — one between your right hand and your partner's left hand and the other between your left and your partner's right.

Exercise: You will each tug back with your right hands, pulling your partner's left hand forward.

Repetitions: Ten to fifteen times.

Benefits: Helps to strengthen and firm the arms, shoulders, and back.

TOWEL TUG 2
(See illus.)

Starting Position: You and your partner sit on the floor facing each other with your legs spread and knees locked tight; the soles of your feet are flat against the soles of your

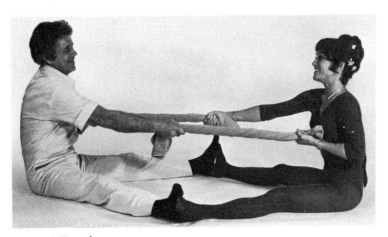

Towel Tug 1

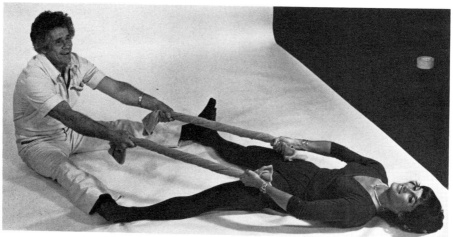

Towel Tug 2

partner's feet. Stretch one towel between your right hand and your partner's left and one between your left and his or her right.

Exercise: You pull all the way back on both towels, bringing your partner forward as you draw back all the way to the floor. Then your partner pulls you up as he or she draws back to the floor.

Repetitions: Eight to ten times.

Benefits: If you keep your abdomen squeezed, this will tone and firm the muscles of the waist and abdomen as well as benefit the shoulders and arms.

TOWEL TUG 3
(See illus.)

Starting Position: Same as for Towel Tugs 1 and 2.

Exercise: In this exercise, you will be forming circles. With the towels pulled taut between you, sway around in a clockwise motion, bringing your torsos as close as possible to the floor in all directions. (As you sway back, you will be pulling your partner forward, and vice versa.) Be sure to keep your abdomens tight as you revolve.

Repetitions: Repeat eight to ten times.

Benefits: Excellent for the abdomen, waist, and arms.

DOUBLE STRETCH
(See illus.)

Starting Position: You and your partner sit on the floor facing each other, holding hands at arm's length. Each of you bend

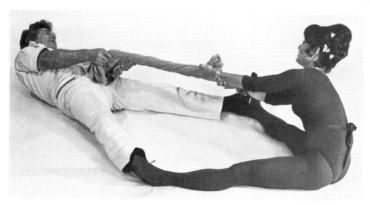

Towel Tug 3

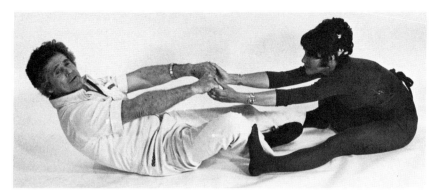

Double Stretch

your right knee, placing your right foot against your left thigh, and extend your left leg so that your left foot braces against your partner's right knee.

Exercise: You pull back as far as you can, pulling your partner forward as you do. Then he or she will pull back, bringing you forward. Keep your abdomen tight and inhale as you pull back and exhale as you are pulled forward. Reverse the position and repeat exercise.

Repetitions: Eight to ten times each position.

Benefits: Stretches you all over and helps to tone the back, abdomen, arms, and legs.

Legs, Hips, and Thighs

BICYCLE FOR TWO
(See illus.)

Starting Position: You and your partner lie down on the floor "foot to foot," at a distance where your toes will be touching if you have your knees bent and your feet flat on the floor. Spread your arms out to your sides to brace yourselves, palms down, and lift your legs so that the soles of your feet meet the soles of your partner's feet.

Exercise: "Bicycle" against each other. Keep your stomach muscles tight, so that you are exercising them while you are working on the legs.

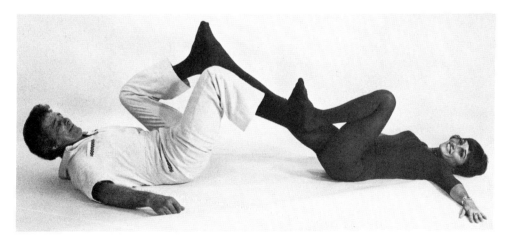

Bicycle for Two

Repetitions: This exercise is so easy that you can probably keep it going for quite a while, but fifteen to twenty cycles is probably sufficient.

Benefits: Helps to tone the legs, hips, and waist.

DOUBLE SWING
(See illus.)

Starting Position: You and your partner lie flat on your backs, head to head. Extend your arms out from your body to brace yourselves, and clasp hands. With your abdomens squeezed, and with your backs flat against the floor, raise your legs straight up in the air toward the ceiling. (If you have a weak back, raise your legs with the knees bent.)

Exercise: You will each twist first to the right, then to the left, bringing your legs almost to the floor each way. (As you twist to the right, your partner will be twisting to his or her right as well, but it will be to your left.)

Repetitions: Eight to ten times in the beginning.

Benefits: Excellent for the abdomen, hips, and waist.

ANKLE WRESTLE

Starting Position: You and your partner sit on the floor facing each other at a distance that will permit you both to extend your legs almost to their full length. Place your legs together between your partner's legs so your ankles touch. Sit up straight, with your abdomen tucked in tight, and with your arms folded in front of you

Exercise: Your object will be to press your legs outward to separate your partner's legs; your partner's object will be to press inward to keep your legs together. Say "Go," apply the pressure, count to five, and relax. Reverse the procedure with your partner's legs between your legs.

Repetitions: Eight to ten times, each direction.

Benefits: If you do the exercise both ways, you will exercise both the inner and outer thighs.

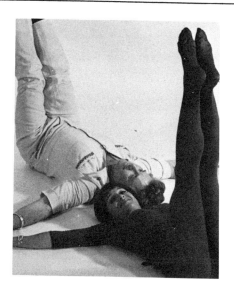 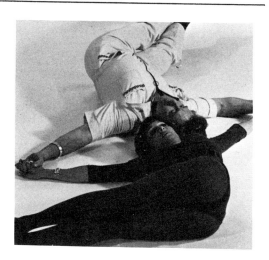

Double Swing

Chapter 13

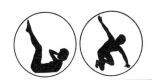

POOL EXERCISES

While you should have your regular daily period of exercise, you do not have to limit yourself to that set 14 minutes a day. If you happen to have a swimming pool, or if you have access to one, you can also get in a bit of exercise while you are relaxing and having fun.

Water is particularly good for exercising, because you get a pressure resistance no matter how you move. And, if you have a weak back, or if you have a problem muscle somewhere, water can be very beneficial; you will be less likely to jerk or snap a muscle or ligament in water.

Of course, if possible, you should do your exercises in warm water rather than cold for the best results. Muscles stretch better and tone better in warm water. (If you have a sore muscle or a torn ligament, you apply cold for the first twenty-four hours after injury, and then heat can be used if the injury is chronic.)

There are many ways to use a pool for exercise; the ones that follow are only a small sample of what you can do. (For example, water volleyball provides excellent exercise, but it does require a group.) I have tried to keep the exercises as simple as possible. Most of them can be done alone in the water. Some require the aid of a volleyball, and some require two volleyballs.

Once you have learned these water exercises, you yourself may be able to come up with others that are equally good. Once your body has become acquainted with the most basic exercises, experiment.

Fundamental Water Exercises

FIGURE EIGHT

Starting Position: Stand at least waist deep in the water and hold on to the side of the pool.

Exercise: Raise your right leg, keeping it straight, and swing it in a circular motion, drawing figure eights with your toes. Shift your weight to your right leg, and draw the figure eights with your left leg.

Repetitions: Eight to ten times each leg.

Benefits: Good for the legs, thighs, and hips.

LEG SWING

Starting Position: Stand at least waist deep in the water, place your feet together, and support yourself with your right hand on the bar or the side of the pool.

Exercise: Keeping your stomach tight, swing your left leg forward and back several times, then out to the side several times. Turn to face the other way, supporting yourself with your left hand on the bar or the side of the pool, and repeat the exercise with your right leg.

Repetitions: About five times each direction.

Benefits: Benefits the thighs, buttocks, waist, and abdomen.

Variations:

1. Return to your original position, with your right hand on the bar or the side of the pool. Swing your left leg forward, around to the side, and back, then return to the original position. Repeat five times, then turn to face the other way, supporting yourself with your left hand on the bar or side of the pool, and repeat the exercise with your right leg. This is particularly beneficial to the inner thighs and the buttocks.

2. Turn your back to the side of the pool, placing your arms on the bar for support. Resting your buttocks against the wall, and with your legs straight and pressed tight together, lift both legs approximately one foot off the bottom of the pool. Swing them back and forth, left to right six to eight times. This is particularly beneficial to the waist and hips.

HIP BOBBING

Starting Position: Stand facing the side of the pool, holding on to the bar with both hands. Bring your legs up, knees bent in front of you, so that both feet brace against the side of the pool.

Exercise: You are going to swing your hips up above the water. First swing your right hip up, then down; then swing your left hip up.

Repetitions: Eight to ten times.

Benefits: Excellent for the thighs, waist, and shoulders.

SIDE BEND

Starting Position: Stand facing the side of the pool, holding on to the bar with both hands. Bring your feet up to the side of the pool about 10 inches apart (or a distance that will permit your knees to be outside your arms).

Exercise: Swing your body to the right so that your right knee touches the side of the pool, then swing to the left to touch your left knee to the side.

Repetitions: Repeat eight to ten times.

Benefits: Particularly good for firming the buttocks.

One-Ball Exercises

BALL EIGHT

Starting Position: Stand out away from the side of the pool, at a place deep enough so that the water reaches your chest or shoulders. Stand with both feet on the bottom of the pool, slightly apart. Grasp the volleyball firmly between your hands straight out in front of your body.

Exercise: Move the ball in a circle in to the left side of your body, out again, and in to the right side of your body, and out again. You are forming figure eights with the volleyball on top of the water. Now try to press the ball down halfway into the water as you continue. Reverse the direction.

Repetitons: Ten to fifteen times.

Benefits: Excellent for the upper arms, chest, and shoulders. If you keep your abdomen tucked in and twist slightly as you form your figure eights, it will also benefit your waist and stomach.

Variation: The above figure eights are horizontal or parallel to the surface of the water. You can also form figure eights vertically by pushing the ball down, up, and around in front of you. Stand with both feet on the bottom of the pool, slightly apart, and with the ball clasped between your hands straight out in front of you. Press it down under the water slightly to your left, then let it surface, and then press it down slightly to your right.

DUNK THE BALL

Starting Position: Stand with both feet together on the bottom of the pool, and with the ball clasped between your hands in front of you.

Exercise: Try to push the ball down as deep as you can without losing your grasp on it.

Repetitions: Press it down and up eight to ten times, keeping your stomach muscles in.

Benefits: Good for the abdomen, back, and arms.

WATERBIKE

Starting Position: Place the ball under your left arm and lie down on your right side.

Exercise: Guiding yourself with your right arm, cycle around in a forward circle several times. Reverse, and cycle backwards for the same number of times. Then shift the ball to your right arm, and perform the exercise for the other side.

Repetitions: Eight or ten times each direction.

Benefits: Good for the thighs and abdominal muscles.

NUTCRACKER

Starting Position: You may not be able to get deeper than your waist for this one. Place the ball between your thighs.

Exercise: Press against the ball with your thighs for a count of five. Then release.

Repetitions: Ten to fifteen times.

Benefits: Helps to firm the thighs and buttocks.

CHARLIE CHAPLIN

Starting Position: Stand in the water with the ball pressed between your thighs.

Exercise: Shuffle flat-footed across the pool. Remember to keep your buttocks tight and your stomach muscles tucked in. You are doing the Charlie Chaplin walk.

Repetitions: In the beginning walk across the pool and back two times. Increase gradually up to five times.

Benefits: Very good for the thighs, buttocks, hips, and waist.

Two-Ball Exercise

CAN-CAN

Starting Position: Stand in the pool at a depth where the water is a few inches below shoulder level. Tuck one ball under each arm.

Exercise: Do the can-can, kicking the right leg up out of the water while the left remains on the bottom of the pool. Return the right to the bottom of the pool, and kick the left up out of the water.

Repetitions: Ten to fifteen times.

Benefits: Good for the hips, waist, buttocks, and legs.

THE SWING

Starting Position: With one ball tucked under each arm, and keeping your back vertical, extend your legs straight out in front of you, keeping them tight together.

Exercise: Once your legs are at a 90-degree angle to your body, bend your knees up to your chest, then down and back behind you. Swing them forward and out in front of you again.

Repetitions: Eight to ten times.

Benefits: A good all-over exercise, but particularly beneficial to the hips, thighs, and buttocks.

THE ESTHER WILLIAMS

Starting Position: With one ball under each arm, allow your body to float on top of the water. (Your legs will not float naturally, you will have to use some effort.)

Exercise: Begin with your legs straight out and together, then bend your right knee, keeping your left leg straight, and swing your right knee over your left thigh. Your right hip will bob up to the surface as you twist. Then swing your right leg back out straight, and swing your left knee over your right thigh. Remember to keep your stomach in.

Repetitions: Fifteen to twenty times.

Benefits: An excellent toner for the waist, hips, and thighs.

SCISSORS

Starting Position: With one ball under each arm, and with your torso vertical, lift your legs to a horizontal position. Keep your stomach muscles in, and keep your legs tight together as you lift them from the hips.

Exercise: When your legs are at a 90-degree angle to your body, spread your legs apart and then back together in a scissorlike motion.

Repetitions: Ten to fifteen times.

Benefits: Particularly good for the inner thighs.

PART IV

THE LA COSTA MENU COOKBOOK

Chapter 14

PREPARING FOOD

The ability to cook low-calorie gourmet food can be an exciting and rewarding accomplishment. Many of the dishes found in the recipe section (Chapter 16) are truly gourmet, delicious, and tempting. Using these recipes can be the beginning of a new approach to cooking and food preparation and will create an awareness of the wonderful natural flavors of foods.

In the preparation of low-calorie yet nutritious meals, there are many cooking tips that can be used to help you skim off excess, unwanted calories from *any* recipe you choose. The end result will still be a meal to be proud of and will be relished by your family and guests alike.

In traditional cooking, fats serve two purposes: they add flavor, and they serve as a preservative for keeping food fresh. Americans have long enjoyed the flavor of fat, as evidenced by the large percentage of fat in the American diet today. The appetite for fat is an acquired tendency and is often seen in infancy and in young children, for even today many parents have the mistaken impression that a fat or overfed baby is a healthy one.

As a preservative, fat at one time was extremely important. Storing food for a long time was almost impossible. Today, with the convenience of refrigeration and freezing methods, storage is no problem. Likewise, the distribution of food is so adequate today that almost any food you desire can be purchased fresh at any time of the year. This makes it possible to cook and serve delicious, fresh, nutritious foods almost immediately with little loss of flavor or quality.

Dressings and Sauces

As I indicated earlier in discussing the fat exchanges in Chapter 5, the dressings we should strive to use are the thin vinegar-and-oil or lemon dressings. Most of the thicker dressings are made with either a mayonnaise or a sour cream base and are extremely high in fat calories. You can, however, produce a thick dressing, sauce, or dip with a lower fat content by substituting low-fat cottage cheese that has been whipped in a blender. The resulting texture and flavor are almost identical to those of the higher-calorie dressing. The additon of a small amount of low-fat yogurt adds tartness if desired.

Whipped low-fat cottage cheese is delicious as a vegetable dip with the addition of onion powder, a little garlic, and some chopped clams. It can also be used in a chicken or tuna salad instead of mayonnaise.

An excellent low-calorie Roquefort dressing can be made using low-fat cottage cheese and a small portion of blue cheese whipped in a blender. Whipped low-fat cottage cheese or cottage cheese whipped with yogurt is delicious on a baked potato in place of butter and sour cream. A very satisfactory Russian or Thousand Island dressing can be made by whipping cottage cheese with diet ketchup (which is salt free and sugar free). You can also make an excellent cocktail sauce from diet ketchup. (Recipes for these dressings are found in Chapter 16.)

Chinese sweet and sour sauce is fairly high in calories because it is made from pineapple juice, brown sugar, cornstarch, and vinegar. An acceptable substitute can be made with unsweetened fruit juice and vinegar. The sauce can be thickened with vegetable gum, which is a noncaloric thickener made from seaweed. Vegetable gums are also known as alginates, and there are many kinds, including gum arabic, gum tragacanth, and gum acacia. These products are usually found in a drug store.

Sautéing

Butter and fat have always been considered indispensable in sautéing and browning meat and vegetables, but there are alternatives to adding all of those extra calories. Many vegetables contain enough natural sugar to brown without adding any fats at all to a sauté pan. Onion is a good example; sliced onions brown beautifully in a hot, dry skillet. Other vegetables may require a little added moisture in the form of beef or chicken stock or wine. When cooking with wine, allow the liquid to boil, thus causing the alcohol (and its calories) to evaporate in the air.

The pan you select for cooking low-fat dishes is very important. Any coated pan with a nonstick surface (such as Teflon) is excellent. A noncaloric vegetable spray can be used with a regular pan and is very good as a substitute for oil. Meats can also be browned to perfection in an ungreased hot skillet; the meat is seared and tenderized just as well as in a heavily oiled pan.

One of the keys to low-calorie food preparation is cooking quickly at high temperatures. Cooking with a wok is one good method. Food prepared without added fat will not be of high quality for long periods. Fat does help to seal juices into foods during storage and during long cooking periods. Therefore, without added fat, foods should be prepared and served as quickly as possible.

Decalorizing a Recipe

After you have tried the recipes in this book, you will enjoy devising low-calorie recipes of your own, or seeing how you can take the extra calories out of some of your standards and cookbook favorites. Ingredients which add unnecessary calories are thickeners (such as flour, cornstarch, or arrowroot), breadings, butter, oils, shortenings, sugar, cream, and sour cream. In some cases, other foods can be substituted, such as vegetable gum for flour, or artificial sweetener for sugar. Many times, all you need do is omit the ingredient you don't want. Try addding herbs and spices or lemon juice to dishes while eliminating salt in all its forms.

To show how to decalorize a standard recipe, let us take the example of a pot roast. Normally a pot roast is rolled in seasoned flour, seared quickly in oil to retain the juices, and then cooked slowly with a lid for a long time. Finally, it is taken out of the oven and the gravy is thickened with flour. To decalorize this recipe, simply sear the pot roast in a preheated dry pan which has been sprayed with a noncaloric vegetable spray. Season the roast with unsalted defatted beef broth, onion powder, garlic, and any other herbs you like. Cook the covered pot roast until tender. Remove the meat and keep the roast warm. The sauce can be thickened by a method called reduction. Simmer the meat juices, uncovered, to evaporate excess water. The sauce thickens on its own and will not give the starchy, pasty texture and flavor of added thickeners. By simply eliminating the oil and flour, you have saved *over 600* excess calories.

Another example is a roast chicken. Any standard recipe will tell you to rub the raw chicken with butter, season with salt, and baste frequently while roasting to brown the bird. An alternative method is to roast the chicken without adding any extra fat. Season the chicken with paprika and garlic powder. Roast it on a bed of aromatic vegetables: sliced carrots, celery, and onions. The vegetables serve two purposes: they add flavor and moisture to the chicken, and they keep the bird from soaking in its own fat — all the melted chicken fat will accumulate under the vegetables. This method can also be utilized when preparing roast veal or beef.

Low-Calorie Hors d'Ouevres

Snack foods are a downfall for many of the best-intentioned dieters. Olives, nuts, potato chips, and dips at cocktail parties seem to be as tempting as the most luscious of desserts, and many times higher in calories. Fortunately, many hostesses now realize that some of their guests may be restricting their intake of calories, and they are offering low-calorie alternatives to the typical high-calorie hors d'ouevres. Sliced fresh raw vegetables such as celery, carrots, radishes, broccoli, cauliflower, and asparagus can look just as tempting as potato chips and are much more nutritious. You probably try to get the most for your money when you purchase a dress or suit, so why not try to get the most for your calories by choosing foods that offer a high percent of vitamins and minerals? Vegetables can be served with a whipped cottage cheese dip or with our Spa Cocktail Sauce (page 222).

Cutting and Trimming Meat

Americans since the first Thanksgiving have used beef, poultry, or fish as the primary food for almost every meal. I can't over emphasize that variety (and this includes meat) in foods makes dining a very pleasant experience. Since portion size and weight of servings are extremely important in controlling your intake of calories, you should have a scale that weighs in grams and ounces in the kitchen to ensure that you are getting the proper amount allowable on your food plan.

Many of us today buy pre-cut and plastic-wrapped meat from the supermarket because it is more convenient. Before cooking your meat and chops, you must trim off all the visible fat that you possibly can. Somewhere in the city in which you live I am sure you can find a butcher who does his own meat cutting and will be happy to please you by preparing and trimming your order exactly as you want it. A good butcher not only will trim meat to your specifications but will weigh and wrap it for you. Buy the leanest meats available with all visible fat removed — this is a rule we cannot neglect.

LAMB:

If you are serving a number of people, you may want to purchase a rack of lamb; if you do, have your butcher defat it for you or defat it yourself. For only one or two persons, two lamb chops each is a routine serving. The ordinary serving of two lamb chops before they are defatted is 360 grams or approximately 12 ounces. Once these two chops have had the fat removed, the weight is 120 grams — almost 8 ounces of fat has been removed. You will be serving 4 ounces of lamb. Broiling is a fine way to cook lamb chops.

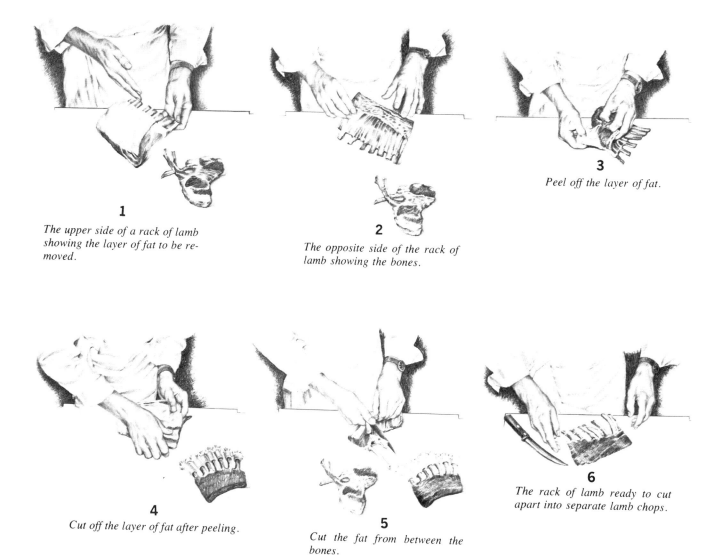

1
The upper side of a rack of lamb showing the layer of fat to be removed.

2
The opposite side of the rack of lamb showing the bones.

3
Peel off the layer of fat.

4
Cut off the layer of fat after peeling.

5
Cut the fat from between the bones.

6
The rack of lamb ready to cut apart into separate lamb chops.

TENDERLOIN STEAK:

Unless you are giving a dinner party, or have a large family, you may not want to purchase a whole tenderloin. However, from a tenderloin strip you can cut a number of smaller steaks even after it has been frozen. It is good to know how to trim a tenderloin strip if the need arises because from it you can easily get ten or twelve 3-ounce steaks and have several pieces of meat which can be used for stew, pot roast, or beef stroganoff.

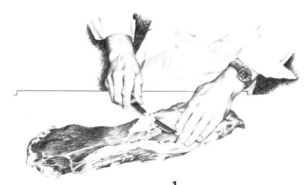

1

The tenderloin of beef showing the thin veil of fat. Cut gently through the veil without cutting into the steak, and peel off.

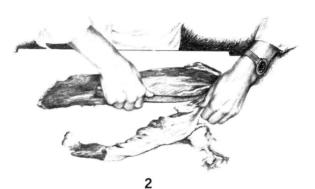

2

Running along the other side of the tenderloin is a strip of very heavy, fatty meat. Remove by using the knife to cut a groove and pull the strip away with your free hand.

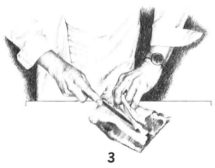

3

Remove the top of the tenderloin which is too tough to serve as steak, and use for stroganoff or stew.

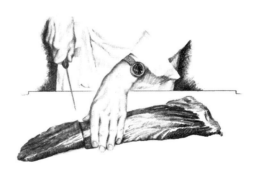

4

Cut the tenderloin into three-ounce steaks, approximately one-inch thick, which are 90 calories each. (After cooking they will be two-ounce steaks.)

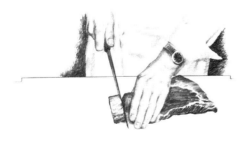

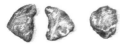

CHICKEN:

The chicken entrées that are included in the menus call for chicken breasts. If you are willing to bone and disjoint a chicken yourself, I advise you to purchase a whole 2- to 2⅓-pound chicken, which will yield serving sizes appropriate for this diet program. Whole chickens are usually fresher than already cut parts, and the chicken carcass left over will make an excellent chicken stock.

If you cannot or do not want to do this, it is best to buy chicken breasts (which any market carries), which are the leanest part of a chicken. Most of the fat in this area lies just under the skin, so the skin and all visible fat must be removed before cooking. Whether or not you prefer the chicken breast with all bone removed is up to you. The bones do not increase the calorie count but they do make eating it a little more difficult.

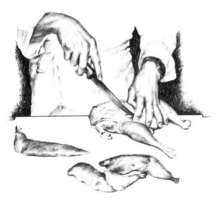

1

Remove the chicken wings, then remove the chicken leg cutting above the thigh, and separate the thigh bone from its socket.

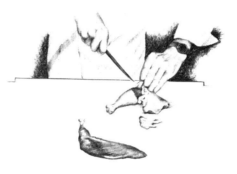

2

Remove the fatty skin from the chicken leg.

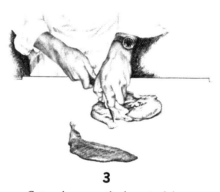

3

Cut and remove the breast of the chicken.

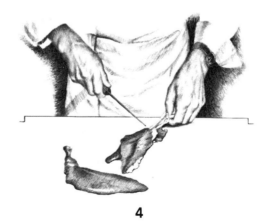

4

Remove the skin from the breast.

Chapter 15

THE MENU PLAN

Breakfast Menu

Calories per Serving:

40	1 Fruit Exchange
68	1 Bread Exchange
40	Puffed Rice (1 oz.)
30	Puffed Wheat (1 oz.)
80	Shredded Wheat (1 oz.)
40	Skim Milk (4 oz.)
73	1 Meat Exchange (1 oz.)
10	Diet Jam (1 tsp.)
45	1 Fat Exchange

Suggestions for Breakfast:

68	1 Slice of Toast
73	1 Egg
40	¼ Canteloupe
80	8 ounces nonfat Milk
___	
261	

OR

40	4 ounces Orange Juice
68	½ cup Cooked Cereal
40	4 ounces Skim Milk
73	1 Egg
45	1 tsp. Margarine
___	
266	

OR

146	2-ounce Breakfast Steak (3 oz. raw wt.)
40	½ Grapefruit
68	1 Slice of Toast
10	1 tsp. Diet Jam
___	
264	

OR

73	¼ cup Low-fat Cottage Cheese
40	1 ounce Puffed Rice
40	4 ounces Nonfat Milk
68	½ Bagel
45	1 tsp. Margarine
___	
266	

DAY 1

Luncheon Menu

Appetizer

30 Cucumber Slices in Yogurt
     with Chives
22 Consommé with Celery Leaves
20 Vegetable Juice Cocktail

Salad

16 Tomato Princesse
16 Hearts of Romaine

Entrée

200 Linguini with Clam Sauce
146 Stuffed Bell Pepper
146 Halibut in Wine Sauce
146 Cottage Cheese Fruit Plate

Vegetable

16 Hot Cabbage Wedges
16 Bean Sprouts with Mushrooms

Dessert

40 Pumpkin Custard
40 Hot Apricot Compote
40 Fresh Grapes

LUNCHEON:	Calories Allowed
800-Calorie Diet 1 appetizer, 1 salad, 1 entrée, 1 vegetable, 1 dessert	260
1000 1 appetizer, 1 salad, 1 entrée, 1 bread exchange, 1 vegetable, 1 dessert	365
1200 1 appetizer, 1 salad, 1 entrée, 1 bread exchange, 1 fat exchange, 1 vegetable, 1 dessert	410

Dinner Menu

Appetizer

40 Fresh Pear Nectar
50 Vegetable Soup
40 Tropical Fruit Supreme

Salad

36 Citrus Bouquet Salad
25 Italian Salad Bowl

Entrée

146 Roast Duck
146 Medallion of Veal Princesse
146 Lobster Ambassador
146 Paprika Chicken

Vegetable

36 Fresh Artichoke with Hot Dip
30 Toasted Potato Shell with Chives
16 Ratatouille

Dessert

40 Coupe St. Jacques
40 Frozen Strawberry Yogurt
40 Hot Apple Compote

DINNER:	Calories Allowed
800-Calorie Diet 1 appetizer, 1 salad, 1 entrée, 1 vegetable, 1 dessert	276
1000 1 appetizer, 1 salad, 1 entée, 1 bread exchange, 1 vegetable, 1 dessert	376
1200 1 appetizer, 1 salad, double entrée, 1 bread exchange, 1 vegetable, 1 dessert	522

DAY 2

Luncheon Menu

Appetizer

25   Consommé of Tomato Soup
40   Broiled Grapefruit
20   Strawberries Supreme

Salad

16   Cabbage Vinaigrette
25   Apple Celery Salad

Entrée

200   Tostada
146   Fluffy Creole Omelette
146   Poached Salmon Americaine
146   Tuna Salad Plate

Vegetable

16   Diced Zucchini Squash
36   Peas and Carrots

Dessert

40   Lemon Gelatin
40   Frozen Blueberry Yogurt
40   Hot Spiced Red Plums

LUNCHEON:	Calories Allowed
800-Calorie Diet	
1 appetizer, 1 salad, 1 entrée, 1 vegetable, 1 dessert	260
1000	
1 appetizer, 1 salad, 1 entrée, 1 bread exchange, 1 vegetable, 1 dessert	365
1200	
1 appetizer, 1 salad, 1 entrée, 1 bread exchange, 1 fat exchange, 1 vegetable, 1 dessert	410

Dinner Menu

Appetizer

50   Seafood Cocktail
25   Beef Broth with Sherry
40   Pineapple Juice Supreme

Salad

16   Hearts of Romaine
20   Green Beans, Sweet Red Peppers, Scallions, and Boston Lettuce

Entrée

146   Roast Leg of Lamb
146   Swiss Steak
146   Trout Capri
146   Broiled Lobster Tail

Vegetable

20   Spinach in Red Wine
36   Julienne of Rutabaga

Dessert

40   Whipped Banana Pudding
40   Ambrosia
40   Boysenberry Parfait

DINNER:	Calories Allowed
800-Calorie Diet	
1 appetizer, 1 salad, 1 entrée, 1 vegetable, 1 dessert	276
1000	
1 appetizer, 1 salad, 1 entrée, 1 bread exchange, 1 vegetable, 1 dessert	376
1200	
1 appetizer, 1 salad, double entrée, 1 bread exchange, 1 vegetable, 1 dessert	522

DAY 3

Luncheon Menu

Appetizer

22 Chicken Broth with Dill
40 Chilled Blueberry Soup
20 Canton Melon Balls

Salad

25 Apple Cabbage Salad
30 Cucumber Slices in Yogurt
     with Chives

Entrée

200 Cobb Salad Bowl
146 Salisbury Steak with Mushrooms
146 Halibut Jardiniere
146 Cold Chicken with Fruit Salad

Vegetable

26 Diced Celery and Carrots
16 Celery Julienne with Pimiento

Dessert

40 Frozen Banana Orange Yogurt
40 Coconut Custard
40 Hot Spiced Peaches

LUNCHEON:	Calories Allowed
800-Calorie Diet 1 appetizer, 1 salad, 1 entrée, 1 vegetable, 1 dessert	260
1000 1 appetizer, 1 salad, 1 entrée, 1 bread exchange, 1 vegetable, 1 dessert	365
1200 1 appetizer, 1 salad, 1 entrée, 1 bread exchange, 1 fat exchange, 1 vegetable, 1 dessert	410

Dinner Menu

Appetizer

40 Tropical Fruit Supreme
40 Fresh Grapefruit Juice
22 Consommé with Hot Peppers

Salad

16 Mixed Green Salad
25 Bean Sprouts, Scallions and
     Water Chestnuts

Entrée

146 Curry of Lamb
146 Broiled Salmon Steak
146 Chicken Cacciatore
146 Roast Sirloin of Beef au Naturel

Vegetable

25 Baked Tomato Parmesan
16 Zucchini Provençale

Dessert

40 Hot Baked Apple
40 Pineapple Apricot Sherbet
40 Lemon Gelatin

DINNER:	Calories Allowed
800-Calorie Diet 1 appetizer, 1 salad, 1 entrée, 1 vegetable, 1 dessert	276
1000 1 appetizer, 1 salad, 1 entrée, 1 bread exchange, 1 vegetable, 1 dessert	376
1200 1 appetizer, 1 salad, double entrée, 1 bread exchange, 1 vegetable, 1 dessert	522

DAY 4

Luncheon Menu

Appetizer

25   Jellied Tomato Consommé
40   Cold Apple Soup
50   Manhattan Clam Chowder

Salad

16   Cauliflower Vinaigrette
25   Iceberg Lettuce Mimosa

Entrée

200   Chicken in the Pot
146   Crab Meat New Orleans
146   London Broil with Mushrooms
146   Chef's Salad Bowl

Vegetable

16   Chopped Spinach
16   Diced Zucchini Squash

Dessert

40   Fresh Orange Juice Gelatin
40   Buttermilk Sherbet
40   Apricot Parfait

Dinner Menu

Appetizer

50   Seafood Cocktail
40   Fresh Fruit Cup
22   Bouillon with Asparagus Tips

Salad

20   Green Beans, Sweet Red Peppers,
       Scallions, and Boston Lettuce
16   Marinated Tomato Salad

Entrée

146   Tenderloin of Beef Stroganoff
146   Broiled Sole with Curried
       Horseradish
146   Scampi Provençale
146   Veal Cutlets

Vegetable

16   Hungarian Brussels Sprouts
20   Cabbage with Sweet Peppers

Dessert

40   Frozen Strawberry Yogurt
40   Fresh Pineapple Wedge
40   Prune Whip

LUNCHEON	Calories Allowed
800-Calorie Diet 1 appetizer, 1 salad, 1 entrée, 1 vegetable, 1 dessert	260
1000 1 appetizer, 1 salad, 1 entrée, 1 bread exchange, 1 vegetable, 1 dessert	365
1200 1 appetizer, 1 salad, 1 entrée, 1 bread exchange, 1 fat exchange, 1 vegetable, 1 dessert	410

DINNER:	Calories Allowed
800-Calorie Diet 1 appetizer, 1 salad, 1 entrée, 1 vegetable, 1 dessert	276
1000 1 appetizer, 1 salad, 1 entrée, 1 bread exchange, 1 vegetable, 1 dessert	376
1200 1 appetizer, 1 salad, double entrée, 1 bread exchange, 1 vegetable, 1 dessert	522

DAY 5

Luncheon Menu

Appetizer

40 Broiled Grapefruit
30 Consommé Carmen
20 Vegetable Juice Cocktail

Salad

25 Apple Celery Salad
25 Bean Sprouts, Scallions, and Water Chestnuts

Entrée

200 Linguini with Clam Sauce
146 Fluffy Creole Omelette
146 Spring Chicken with Lemon and Ginger
146 Cold Sockeye Salmon Plate

Vegetable

16 Green Beans Italienne
25 Baked Tomato Parmesan

Dessert

40 Hot Spiced Peaches
40 Coconut Custard
40 Frozen Blueberry Yogurt

Dinner Menu

Appetizer

50 Vegetable Soup
50 Shrimp Cocktail
20 Canton Melon Balls

Salad

16 Mixed Green Salad
16 Coleslaw

Entrée

146 Broiled Lobster Tail
146 Roast Leg of Lamb
146 Paprika Chicken
146 Poached Flounder

Vegetable

36 Mixed Vegetables
16 Parsleyed Cauliflower

Dessert

40 Boysenberry Parfait
40 Ambrosia
40 Pineapple Apricot Sherbet

LUNCHEON:	Calories Allowed
800-Calorie Diet 1 appetizer, 1 salad, 1 entrée, 1 vegetable, 1 dessert	260
1000 1 appetizer, 1 salad, 1 entrée, 1 bread exchange, 1 vegetable, 1 dessert	365
1200 1 appetizer, 1 salad, 1 entrée, 1 bread exchange, 1 fat exchange, 1 vegetable, 1 dessert	410

DINNER:	Calories Allowed
800-Calorie Diet 1 appetizer, 1 salad, 1 entrée, 1 vegetable, 1 dessert	276
1000 1 appetizer, 1 salad, 1 entrée, 1 bread exchange, 1 vegetable, 1 dessert	376
1200 1 appetizer, 1 salad, double entrée, 1 bread exchange, 1 vegetable, 1 dessert	522

DAY 6

Luncheon Menu

Appetizer

25   Iced Gazpacho
40   Boysenberry Juice
22   Chicken Broth with Dill

Salad

25   Fresh Spinach Salad
16   Celery Vinaigrette

Entrée

146   London Broil with Mushrooms
146   Halibut Jardiniere
146   Chef's Salad Bowl
146   Fruit Plate with Cottage Cheese

Vegetable

16   Asparagus Spears
36   Hot Spiced Beets

Dessert

40   Hot Baked Apple
40   Pumpkin Custard
40   Frozen Pineapple Slices

LUNCHEON:	Calories Allowed
800-Calorie Diet 1 appetizer, 1 salad, 1 entrée, 1 vegetable, 1 dessert	260
1000 1 appetizer, 1 salad, 1 entrée, 1 bread exchange, 1 vegetable, 1 dessert	365
1200 1 appetizer, 1 salad, 1 entrée, 1 bread exchange, 1 fat exchange, 1 vegetable, 1 dessert	410

Dinner Menu

Appetizer

50   Lobster Cocktail Supreme
25   Broccoli Potage
40   Fresh Grapefruit Juice

Salad

16   Sliced Tomatoes with Chopped Scallion Tops
25   Boston Lettuce with Avocado

Entrée

146   Chicken Amandine
146   Tenderloin of Beef Stroganoff
146   Broiled Salmon Steak
146   Lamb Shish Kabob

Vegetable

36   French Peas
16   Hungarian Brussels Sprouts

Dessert

40   Hot Baked Pear
40   Whipped Banana Pudding
40   Chocolate Mousse

DINNER:	Calories Allowed
800-Calorie Diet 1 appetizer, 1 salad, 1 entrée 1 vegetable, 1 dessert	276
1000 1 appetizer, 1 salad, 1 entrée, 1 bread exchange, 1 vegetable, 1 dessert	376
1200 1 appetizer, 1 salad, double entrée, 1 bread exchange, 1 vegetable, 1 dessert	522

DAY 7

Luncheon Menu

Appetizer

40 Chilled Blueberry Soup
20 Vegetable Juice Cocktail
50 Manhattan Clam Chowder

Salad

25 Asparagus with Fresh Fruit Dressing
16 Coleslaw

Entrée

200 Tostada
146 Minute Steak
146 Poached Salmon Americaine
146 Sliced Beef Platter Garni

Vegetable

16 Savoy Green Beans
16 Braised Lettuce

Dessert

40 Buttermilk Sherbet
40 Apricot Parfait
40 Fresh Grapes

	Calories Allowed
LUNCHEON:	
800 Calorie Diet	
1 appetizer, 1 salad, 1 entrée, 1 vegetable, 1 dessert	260
1000	
1 appetizer, 1 salad, 1 entrée, 1 bread exchange, 1 vegetable, 1 dessert	365
1200	
1 appetizer, 1 salad, 1 entrée, 1 bread exchange, 1 fat exchange, 1 vegetable, 1 dessert	410

Dinner Menu

Appetizer

40 Broiled Grapefruit
40 Tropical Fruit Supreme
25 Beef Broth au Sherry

Salad

16 Sliced Tomatoes with Fines Herbs
16 Hearts of Romaine with Radishes, Zucchini, and Tomato

Entrée

146 Scampi Provençale
146 Roast Sirloin of Beef au Naturel
146 Chicken Cacciatore
146 Medallion of Veal Princesse

Vegetable

36 Baby Carrots à l'Orange
16 Fresh Broccoli with Lemon

Dessert

40 Hot Apple Compote
40 Fresh Pineapple Wedge
40 Lemon Gelatin

	Calories Allowed
DINNER:	
800-Calorie Diet	
1 appetizer, 1 salad, 1 entrée, 1 vegetable, 1 dessert	276
1000	
1 appetizer, 1 salad, 1 entrée, 1 bread exchange, 1 vegetable, 1 dessert	376
1200	
1 appetizer, 1 salad, double entrée, 1 bread exchange, 1 vegetable, 1 dessert	522

DAY 8

Luncheon Menu

Appetizer

40   Fresh Apple Juice
20   Strawberries Supreme
25   Consommé of Tomato Soup

Salad

16   Cauliflower Vinaigrette
36   Orange Gelatin Salad

Entrée

146   Halibut in Wine Sauce
146   Salisbury Steak with Mushrooms
146   Cold Lobster Platter
146   Fruit Plate with Cottage Cheese

Vegetable

36   Whipped Squash
16   Asparagus Spears

Dessert

40   Apple Juice Frappé
40   Hot Apricot Compote
40   Hot Baked Fresh Pear

Dinner Menu

Appetizer

20   Consommé with Hot Peppers
20   Fresh Grapefruit Sections
25   Jellied Tomato Consommé

Salad

25   La Costa Spa Salad
36   Pickled Beets

Entrée

146   Broiled Sole with Curried
          Horseradish
146   Veal Cutlets
146   Pepper Steak La Costa
146   Coq au Vin

Vegetable

30   Toasted Potato Shell with Chives
16   Mushrooms with Cherry Tomatoes

Dessert

40   Chocolate Mousse
40   Whipped Banana Pudding
40   Fresh Pineapple Yogurt

	Calories Allowed
LUNCHEON:	
800-Calorie Diet	
1 appetizer, 1 salad, 1 entrée, 1 vegetable, 1 dessert	260
1000	
1 appetizer, 1 salad, 1 entrée, 1 bread exchange, 1 vegetable, 1 dessert	365
1200	
1 appetizer, 1 salad, 1 entrée, 1 bread exchange, 1 fat exchange, 1 vegetable, 1 dessert	410

	Calories Allowed
DINNER:	
800-Calorie Diet	
1 appetizer, 1 salad, 1 entrée, 1 vegetable, 1 dessert	276
1000	
1 appetizer, 1 salad, 1 entrée, 1 bread exchange, 1 vegetable, 1 dessert	376
1200	
1 appetizer, 1 salad, double entrée, 1 bread exchange, 1 vegetable, 1 dessert	522

DAY 9

Luncheon Menu

Appetizer

40	Fresh Grapefruit Juice
30	Consommé Carmen
40	Cold Apple Soup

Salad

30	Marinated Crisp Fresh Vegetables
20	Boston Lettuce with Radish and Tomato Slices

Entrée

200	Chicken in the Pot
146	Sweet and Sour Salmon
146	Beef Shish Kabob
146	Tuna Salad Plate

Vegetable

16	Broiled Eggplant Slices
16	Zucchini Provençale

Dessert

40	Pineapple Apricot Sherbet
40	Hot Spiced Peaches
40	Coconut Custard

Dinner Menu

Appetizer

40	Tropical Fruit Supreme
40	Fresh Pear Nectar
25	Broccoli Potage

Salad

125	Fresh Spinach Salad
16	Sliced Tomatoes with Chopped Scallion Tops

Entrée

146	Lobster Ambassador
146	Filet Mignon
146	Paprika Chicken
146	Beef Curry

Vegetable

16	Parsleyed Cauliflower
20	Cabbage with Sweet Red Peppers

Dessert

40	Fresh Pineapple Wedge
40	Prune Whip
40	Frozen Strawberry Yogurt

LUNCHEON:	Calories Allowed
800-Calorie Diet 1 appetizer, 1 salad, 1 entrée, 1 vegetable, 1 dessert	260
1000 1 appetizer, 1 salad, 1 entrée, 1 bread exchange, 1 vegetable, 1 dessert	365
1200 1 appetizer, 1 salad, 1 entrée, 1 bread exchange, 1 fat exchange, 1 vegetable, 1 dessert	410

DINNER:	Calories Allowed
800-Calorie Diet 1 appetizer, 1 salad, 1 entrée, 1 vegetable, 1 dessert	276
1000 1 appetizer, 1 salad, 1 entrée, 1 bread exchange, 1 vegetable, 1 dessert	376
1200 1 appetizer, 1 salad, double entrée, 1 bread exchange, 1 vegetable, 1 dessert	522

DAY 10

Luncheon Menu

Appetizer

22   Consommé with Celery Leaves
40   Apricot Juice
20   Canton Melon Balls

Salad

16   Tomato Princesse
25   Iceberg Lettuce Mimosa

Entrée

146   Poached Salmon Americaine
146   Salisbury Steak with Mushrooms
146   Sliced Beef Platter Garni
146   Cold Chicken with Fruit Salad

Vegetable

16   Sweet and Sour Red Cabbage
25   Yellow Crookneck Squash with
       French Peas

Dessert

40   Hot Baked Apple
40   Fresh Orange Juice Gelatin
40   Frozen Blueberry Yogurt

Dinner Menu

Appetizer

40   Pineapple Juice Supreme
25   Beef Broth au Sherry
50   Shrimp Cocktails

Salad

25   Bean Sprouts, Scallions, and Water
       Chestnuts
16   Hearts of Romaine with Radishes,
       Zucchini, and Tomato

Entrée

146   Roast Duck
146   Roast Sirloin of Beef au Naturel
146   Chicken Cacciatore
146   Poached Flounder

Vegetable

16   Fresh Broccoli with Lemon
36   Julienne of Rutabaga

Dessert

40   Hot Spiced Red Plums
40   Coupe St. Jacques
40   Ambrosia

LUNCHEON:	Calories Allowed
800-Calorie Diet 1 appetizer, 1 salad, 1 entrée, 1 vegetable, 1 dessert	260
1000 1 appetizer, 1 salad, 1 entrée, 1 bread exchange, 1 vegetable, 1 dessert	365
1200 1 appetizer, 1 salad, 1 entrée, 1 bread exchange, 1 fat exchange, 1 vegetable, 1 dessert	410

DINNER:	Calories Allowed
800-Calorie Diet 1 appetizer, 1 salad, 1 entrée, 1 vegetable, 1 dessert	276
1000 1 appetizer, 1 salad, 1 entrée, 1 bread exchange, 1 vegetable, 1 dessert	376
1200 1 appetizer, 1 salad, double entrée, 1 bread exchange, 1 vegetable, 1 dessert	522

DAY 11

Luncheon Menu

Appetizer

25	Iced Gazpacho
20	Vegetable Juice Cocktail
30	Consommé Carmen

Salad

16	Cucumber Vinaigrette
36	Orange Gelatin Salad

Entrée

200	Cobb Salad Bowl
146	Broiled Trout
146	London Broil with Mushrooms
146	Fruit Plate with Cottage Cheese

Vegetable

36	Peas and Carrots
16	Hot Cabbage Wedge

Dessert

40	Apple Juice Frappé
40	Pumpkin Custard
40	Buttermilk Sherbet

Dinner Menu

Appetizer

25	Broccoli Potage
50	Seafood Cocktail
20	Grapefruit Sections

Salad

16	Marinated Tomato Salad
36	Pickled Beets

Entrée

146	Lamb Shish Kabob
146	Pepper Steak La Costa
146	Tenderloin of Beef Stroganoff
146	Medallion of Veal Princesse

Vegetable

36	Baked Hubbard Squash
16	Green Beans with Scallion Tops

Dessert

40	Hot Baked Pear
40	Whipped Banana Pudding
40	Chocolate Mousse

LUNCHEON: Calories Allowed

800-Calorie Diet
1 appetizer, 1 salad, 1 entrée, 1 vegetable, 1 dessert   260

1000
1 appetizer, 1 salad, 1 entrée, 1 bread exchange, 1 vegetable, 1 dessert   365

1200
1 appetizer, 1 salad, 1 entrée, 1 bread exchange, 1 fat exchange, 1 vegetable, 1 dessert   410

DINNER: Calories Allowed

800-Calorie Diet
1 appetizer, 1 salad, 1 entrée, 1 vegetable, 1 dessert   276

1000
1 appetizer, 1 salad, 1 entrée, 1 bread exchange, 1 vegetable, 1 dessert   376

1200
1 appetizer, 1 salad, double entrée, 1 bread exchange, 1 vegetable, 1 dessert   522

DAY 12

Luncheon Menu

Appetizer

40   Apricot Juice
20   Strawberries Supreme
25   Consommé of Tomato Soup

Salad

16   Celery Vinaigrette
25   Apple Cabbage Salad

Entrée

200   Tostada
146   Spring Chicken with
          Lemon and Ginger
146   Cold Lobster Platter
146   Chef's Salad Bowl

Vegetable

16   Savory Green Beans
25   Yellow Crookneck Squash with
          French Peas

Dessert

40   Coconut Custard
40   Hot Spiced Red Plums
40   Frozen Pineapple Slices

Dinner Menu

Appetizer

40   Fresh Fruit Cup
22   Consommé with Hot Peppers
40   Fresh Pear Nectar

Salad

16   Sliced Tomato with Fines Herbs
25   Boston Lettuce with Avocado

Entrée

146   Roast Leg of Lamb
146   Trout Capri
146   Filet Mignon
146   Chicken Amandine

Vegetable

36   French Peas
16   Broiled Eggplant Slices

Dessert

40   Frozen Banana Orange Yogurt
40   Lemon Gelatin
40   Boysenberry Parfait

LUNCHEON:	Calories Allowed
800-Calorie Diet	
1 appetizer, 1 salad, 1 entrée, 1 vegetable, 1 dessert	260
1000	
1 appetizer, 1 salad, 1 entrée, 1 bread exchange, 1 vegetable, 1 dessert	365
1200	
1 appetizer, 1 salad, 1 entrée, 1 bread exchange, 1 fat exchange, 1 vegetable, 1 dessert	410

DINNER:	Calories Allowed
800-Calorie Diet	
1 appetizer, 1 salad, 1 entrée, 1 vegetable, 1 dessert	276
1000	
1 appetizer, 1 salad, 1 entrée, 1 bread exchange, 1 vegetable, 1 dessert	376
1200	
1 appetizer, 1 salad, double entrée, 1 bread exchange, 1 vegetable, 1 dessert	522

DAY 13

Luncheon Menu

Appetizer

40 Fresh Apple Juice
40 Chilled Blueberry Soup
22 Bouillon with Asparagus Tips

Salad

20 Boston Lettuce with Radish and Tomato Slices
16 Cucumber Vinaigrette

Entrée

146 Stuffed Bell Pepper
146 Crab Meat New Orleans
146 Sliced Beef Platter Garni
146 Cold Chicken with Fruit Salad

Vegetable

16 Bean Sprouts with Mushrooms
16 Sweet and Sour Red Cabbage

Dessert

40 Hot Apricot Compote
40 Pumpkin Custard
40 Fresh Grapes

Dinner Menu

Appetizer

50 Shrimp Cocktail
50 Vegetable Soup
40 Pineapple Juice Supreme

Salad

25 Italian Salad Bowl
36 Citrus Bouquet Salad

Entrée

146 Swiss Steak
146 Roast Duck
146 Curry of Lamb
146 Broiled Salmon Steak

Vegetable

16 Braised Lettuce
36 Baked Hubbard Squash

Dessert

40 Prune Whip
40 Fresh Orange Juice Gelatin
40 Buttermilk Sherbet

	Calories Allowed
LUNCHEON:	
800-Calorie Diet — 1 appetizer, 1 salad, 1 entrée, 1 vegetable, 1 dessert	260
1000 — 1 appetizer, 1 salad, 1 entrée, 1 bread exchange, 1 vegetable, 1 dessert	365
1200 — 1 appetizer, 1 salad, 1 entrée, 1 bread exchange, 1 fat exchange, 1 vegetable, 1 dessert	410

	Calories Allowed
DINNER:	
800-Calorie Diet — 1 appetizer, 1 salad, 1 entrée, 1 vegetable, 1 dessert	276
1000 — 1 appetizer, 1 salad, 1 entrée, 1 bread exchange, 1 vegetable, 1 dessert	376
1200 — 1 appetizer, 1 salad, double entrée, 1 bread exchange, 1 vegetable, 1 dessert	522

DAY 14

Luncheon Menu

Appetizer

20   Grapefruit Sections
22   Consommé with Celery Leaves
25   Iced Gazpacho

Salad

16   Cabbage Vinaigrette
25   Asparagus with Fresh Fruit
      Dressing

Entrée

146   Beef Shish Kabob
146   Broiled Trout
146   Minute Steak
146   Cold Sockeye Salmon Plate

Vegetable

16   Celery Julienne with Pimiento
36   Hot Spiced Beets

Dessert

40   Apple Juice Frappé
40   Coupe St. Jacques
40   Fresh Pineapple Yogurt

	Calories Allowed
LUNCHEON:	
800-Calorie Diet 1 appetizer, 1 salad, 1 entrée, 1 vegetable, 1 dessert	260
1000 1 appetizer, 1 salad, 1 entrée, 1 bread exchange, 1 vegetable, 1 dessert	365
1200 1 appetizer, 1 salad, 1 entrée, 1 bread exchange, 1 fat exchange, 1 vegetable, 1 dessert	410

Dinner Menu

Appetizer

50   Lobster Cocktail
22   Chicken Broth with Dill
40   Fresh Fruit Cup

Salad

16   Mixed Green Salad
25   La Costa Salad

Entrée

146   Pepper Steak La Costa
146   Coq au Vin
146   Lamb Shish Kabob
146   Poached Flounder

Vegetable

36   Mixed Vegetables
16   Green Beans with Scallion Tops

Dessert

40   Apricot Parfait
40   Chocolate Mousse
40   Hot Spiced Red Plums

	Calories Allowed
DINNER:	
800-Caolrie Diet 1 appetizer, 1 salad, 1 entrée, 1 vegetable, 1 dessert	276
1000 1 appetizer, 1 salad, 1 entrée, 1 bread exchange, 1 vegetable, 1 dessert	376
1200 1 appetizer, 1 salad, double entrée, 1 bread exchange, 1 vegetable, 1 dessert	522

Chapter 16

THE RECIPES

APPETIZERS

PEAR NECTAR

4 servings of
40 calories each

Ingredients

16 oz. unsweetened pear nectar   2 tsp. lime juice

Method

Combine pear nectar and lime juice. Pour into juice glasses (4 ounces per person) and chill well before serving.

〰〰〰〰〰〰〰〰〰〰〰〰〰

FRESH GRAPEFRUIT JUICE

4 servings of
40 calories each

Ingredients

16 oz. fresh squeezed
   grapefruit juice

Method

Chill the grapefruit juice well before serving.

〰〰〰〰〰〰〰〰〰〰〰〰〰

PINEAPPLE JUICE SUPREME

4 servings of
40 calories each

Ingredients

12 oz. unsweetened pineapple
   juice

Method

Fill juice glasses with the pineapple juice and serve well chilled.

BROILED GRAPEFRUIT

4 servings of
40 calories each

Ingredients

2 medium grapefruits, cut in
half

2 Tbsp. dry sherry

Method

With a grapefruit knife, separate the flesh of the fruit from the shell and separate into sections, making sure they are loosened from the peel. Sprinkle with sherry and broil until the grapefruits are slightly brown and the tops glazed. The alcohol in the sherry evaporates during broiling, so no calories are added.

STRAWBERRIES SUPREME

4 servings of
20 calories each

Ingredients

2 cups fresh strawberries

Method

Serve one-half cup of strawberries per person. May be served with a sprig of fresh mint if desired.

APRICOT JUICE

4 servings of
40 calories each

Ingredients

16 oz. unsweetened apricot
juice

4 lime wedges

Method

Pour into chilled juice glasses 4 ounces per person, and serve a lime wedge as a garnish with each.

FRESH GRAPEFRUIT SECTIONS

4 servings of
20 calories each

Ingredients

1 medium grapefruit

Method

Peel the grapefruit. Remove whole sections from the membrane. Chill well. Garnish with a mint leaf if desired.

SEAFOOD COCKTAIL

4 servings of
50 calories each

Ingredients

2 large prawns, cooked and
   cooled
2 oz. lobster meat, cut into
   bite-size pieces

2 oz. crab meat, cut into
   bite-size pieces
4 lemon wedges
4 Tbsp. Spa Cocktail Sauce

Method

Slice the prawns in half lengthwise. Combine with lobster and crab; arrange in chilled champagne glasses. Serve with Spa Cocktail Sauce (p. 222) and garnish each serving with a lemon wedge.

VEGETABLE JUICE WITH LEMON

4 servings of
20 calories each

Ingredients

16 oz. unsalted vegetable juice

Method

Chill juice well. Serve 4 ounces per person, garnished with a slice of lemon.

CANTON MELON BALLS

4 servings of
20 calories each

Ingredients

2 cups mixed melon balls, in
    season

Method

A combination of melons may be used for this, cantaloupes, honeydew, and crenshaw are a good combination. Garnish with a sprig of fresh mint if desired.

CHILLED BLUEBERRY SOUP

4 servings of
40 calories each

Ingredients

1½ cups unsweetened frozen
    blueberries, thawed
1 cup unsweetened apple juice

1½ cups water
4 thin lemon slices

Method

Blend the apple juice, blueberries, and water in a blender until the blueberries are puréed. Strain and refrigerate covered for one hour. Strain the juices and allow any sediment to settle to the bottom. Skim the top so a clear product will result. Serve in chilled bouillon cups, garnished with a lemon slice, or float several whole berries on top.

SHRIMP COCKTAIL

4 servings of
50 calories each

Ingredients

8 large prawns, cooked and
    cooled
shredded lettuce

4 thin lemon slices
4 Tbsp. Spa Cocktail Sauce

Method

Slice each shrimp in half lengthwise. Place a little shredded lettuce in the bottom of 4 cocktail glasses, top with four shrimp halves per person, and garnish with a lemon slice. Serve with Spa Cocktail Sauce (page 222).

JELLIED TOMATO CONSOMMÉ

4 servings of
25 calories each

Ingredients

6 oz. unsalted tomato juice
2 cups unsalted defatted beef
    broth

3 tsp. plain gelatin, softened in
    a little cold water

Method

Combine all the ingredients, blending well. Pour into a shallow pan and chill thoroughly. Cut the consommé into one-inch cubes and serve in an ice bouillon cup.

LOBSTER COCKTAIL SUPREME

4 servings of
50 calories each

Ingredients

2 3-oz. lobster tails with shell
2 green onions, chopped
1 lemon slice
1 bay leaf

pinch white pepper
2 sprigs fresh parsley
4 Tbsp. Spa Cocktail Sauce

Method

Place the lobster tails on a cutting board and split each tail with a heavy French knife. Fold the tail open, remove the meat, and set aside. Place the empty shells and remaining ingredients in a saucepan along with 2 cups of water. Bring the lobster stock to a boil and simmer for two minutes, uncovered. Remove the shells, bay leaf, and parsley. Place the lobster meat in the hot stock and simmer for 4–5 minutes. Do not overcook. Remove from the heat and allow the lobster meat to cool in the stock. Remove the cooled meat and chill thoroughly.

Just before serving, cut the lobster meat into bite-size pieces and place on a bed of shredded lettuce, garnished with a slice of lemon. Serve with Spa Cocktail Sauce (page 222).

ICED GAZPACHO

4 servings of
25 calories each

Ingredients

1 small zucchini

2 Tbsp. chopped chives

½ green pepper, seeded and
    diced
1 cucumber, diced
2 small tomatoes, diced
½ jalapeño pepper, seeded and
    diced

½ clove garlic, minced
pinch granulated garlic
1 cup unsalted tomato juice
½ cup beef bouillon

Method

Place all the ingredients into a blender and blend for a few seconds or until the vegetables are chopped finely. Chill well. Serve in chilled soup cups.

~~~~~~

FRESH APPLE JUICE

4 servings of
40 calories each

Ingredients

2 medium golden delicious
    apples

1 tsp. lemon juice

Method

Peel and core the apples. Cut into small pieces and place in a blender. Blend the apples into a fine purée, adding the lemon juice to prevent them from turning brown. Chill thoroughly and serve in chilled juice glasses.

~~~~~~

COLD APPLE SOUP

6 servings of
40 calories each

Ingredients

1 small yellow or green apple
1 cup unsweetened apple juice
1 cup fresh orange juice,
    strained

1 cup water

Method

Wash, core, and slice the apple into small strips. Do not peel. Combine the apple juice and orange juice with the sliced apples. Allow the apples and juice to chill. Chill thoroughly. Serve in chilled soup cups.

CITRUS BOUQUET SALAD

4 servings of
36 calories each

Ingredients

12 grapefruit sections
12 orange sections

crisp lettuce cups
4 Tbsp. Spa French Dressing

Method

Arrange grapefruit and orange sections alternately in the lettuce cups. Serve with Spa French Dressing (page 183).

FRESH FRUIT CUP

4 servings of
40 calories each

Ingredients

4 oz. melon, diced
1 small orange, peeled and
    sectioned

½ cup fresh strawberries,
    sliced
2 Tbsp. fresh orange juice

Method

Combine the fresh fruits, and cover with orange juice. Portion into chilled champagne glasses and serve well chilled.

FRESH ORANGE JUICE GELATIN

4 servings of
40 calories each

Ingredients

2 cups freshly squeezed orange
    juice
¼ cup warm water

1½ tsp. plain gelatin
grated orange rind

Method

Soften the gelatin in warm water. Combine the orange juice and gelatin and refrigerate until jelled. Cut the gelatin into small cubes and serve in champagne glasses. Garnish with grated orange rind.

TROPICAL FRUIT SUPREME

6 servings of
40 calories each

Ingredients

1 small papaya, peeled and
 diced
1 small mango, peeled and
 sliced

¼ small pineapple, diced

Method

Combine fruits and chill well. Serve in champagne glasses with a sprig of mint as a garnish.

SOUPS

CHICKEN BROTH WITH DILL

4 servings of
22 calories each

Ingredients

4 cups unsalted defatted
chicken broth

pinch dill

Method

Heat the chicken broth and dill together. Serve hot in bouillon cups.

BEEF BROTH AU SHERRY

4 servings of
22 calories each

Ingredients

4 cups unsalted defatted beef
broth

1 Tbsp. dry sherry

Method

Combine beef broth and sherry. Heat uncovered to allow the alcohol to evaporate. Serve hot in bouillon cups.

CONSOMMÉ WITH CELERY LEAVES

3 servings of
22 calories each

Ingredients

3 cups unsalted defatted beef
broth
pinch whole celery seeds

dash white pepper
inner leaves of 3 celery stalks,
chopped

Method

Add the celery seeds and pepper to the broth and heat. Just before serving, add the chopped celery leaves. Serve very hot in bouillon cups.

BROCCOLI POTAGE

4 servings of
25 calories each

Ingredients

3 cups unsalted defatted
    chicken broth
8 oz. fresh broccoli, cut into
    small pieces

dash white pepper

Method

Bring the chicken broth to a boil and add the broccoli and pepper. Bring the liquid back to a boil and cook until broccoli is tender. Cool slightly and purée in a blender. Reheat before serving; ladle into hot bouillon cups.

VEGETABLE SOUP

4 servings of
50 calories each

Ingredients

3 cups unsalted, defatted beef
    broth
2 Tbsp. finely chopped carrot
4 cauliflower buds, chopped
1 medium tomato, peeled and
    diced

½ cup diced rutabaga
½ cup green peas
white pepper to taste

Method

Combine all ingredients and simmer covered for 25–30 minutes. Garnish with fresh chopped chives if desired. Serve hot in bouillon cups.

BOUILLON WITH ASPARAGUS TIPS

4 servings of
25 calories each

Ingredients

4 cups unsalted, defatted beef
    broth

½ cup asparagus tips

Method

Combine the broth and asparagus and simmer, covered, until the asparagus is tender. Serve hot in bouillon cups.

MANHATTAN CLAM CHOWDER

3 servings of
50 calories each

Ingredients

6 oz. chopped clams, with
    juice
1 small tomato, seeded and
    chopped
8 oz. unsalted tomato juice
¼ green pepper, seeded and
    diced

1 tsp. diced green onion
1 bay leaf
¼ tsp. whole thyme
juice of ¼ lemon
½ cup water

Method

Drain clams, reserving juice. Combine clam juice and remaining ingredients.
Simmer, covered, until vegetables are tender. Add the chopped clams and heat
through. Serve very hot in bouillon cups.

CONSOMMÉ CARMEN

4 servings of
30 calories each

Ingredients

3½ cups unsalted, defatted
    beef broth
1 medium tomato, peeled and
    diced

¼ cup cooked rice

Method

Heat the broth. Add the chopped tomato and the cooked rice. Serve very hot in
bouillon cups.

CONSOMMÉ OF TOMATO SOUP

5 servings of
25 calories each

Ingredients

2 oz. unsalted tomato paste
2 Tbsp. dietetic tomato
    ketchup
1 cup unsalted, defatted beef
    broth

2 bay leaves
white pepper to taste
1 medium tomato, peeled,
    seeded, and chopped

Method

Combine all ingredients except the tomato and simmer in a pot for 15 minutes. Blend the chopped tomato into the soup and simmer 5 more minutes. Serve very hot.

∞∞∞∞∞∞∞∞∞∞∞∞∞∞∞∞∞∞∞∞∞∞∞∞∞∞

CONSOMMÉ WITH HOT PEPPERS

4 servings of
22 calories each

Ingredients

4 cups unsalted, defatted beef broth

½ yellow chili pepper, seeded and chopped

½ green sweet pepper, seeded and chopped

Method

Combine all ingredients and heat thoroughly. Portion into hot bouillon cups and garnish with chives if desired.

∞∞∞∞∞∞∞∞∞∞∞∞∞∞∞∞∞∞∞∞∞∞∞∞∞∞

CHICKEN CONSOMME

8–10 servings of
25 calories each

Ingredients

1 3-lb. whole chicken
2½ quarts unsalted, defatted chicken broth or water
1 onion, sliced
2 leeks, sliced

2 carrots, sliced
3 stalks celery, sliced
8 parsley stems and stalks
8 whole peppercorns, crushed

Method

Put chicken into Dutch oven or stock pot and cover with remaining ingredients. Bring to a boil, skimming occasionally until chicken is tender. Remove chicken, cool, and debone. Return skin, bones, and scraps to broth and simmer, covered, for one hour. Strain broth and chill overnight to allow fat to come to the surface. When ready to use, remove solidified fat from surface and reheat.

SALADS

BOSTON LETTUCE WITH RADISH AND TOMATO

4 servings of
20 calories each

Ingredients

1 head Boston lettuce
4 red radishes, sliced

1 small tomato, quartered

Method

Wash and cut the Boston lettuce into quarters. Garnish with the radishes and tomato. Serve with favorite Spa salad dressing.

CABBAGE VINAIGRETTE

4 servings of
16 calories each

Ingredients

2 cups shredded cabbage
Spa Vinaigrette Dressing

endive

Method

Combine cabbage and enough Spa Vinaigrette Dressing (page 182) to cover. Marinate refrigerated for 2–3 hours. Remove the cabbage with a slotted spoon and serve on a bed of endive.

SLICED TOMATOES WITH CHOPPED SCALLIONS

4 servings of
16 calories each

Ingredients

2 medium tomatoes, washed,
  dried, and sliced

endive hearts
1 scallion, chopped

Method

Arrange the tomato slices on a bed of endive hearts and sprinkle with the scallions. Serve with a Spa salad dressing.

MIXED GREEN SALAD

4 servings of
16 calories each

Ingredients

½ head iceberg lettuce   1 bunch fresh watercress
½ head hearts of romaine

Method

Tear lettuce into bite-size pieces and toss gently. Crisp in chopped ice. When crisp, drain and dry the greens. Serve on chilled salad plates.

ASPARAGUS WITH FRESH FRUIT DRESSING

4 servings of
25 calories each

Ingredients

12 large stalks asparagus,   1 small apple, chopped fine
   cooked and chilled   1 tsp. lemon juice
4 Tbsp. chopped melon   artificial sweetener to taste
4 large fresh strawberries   (optional)

Method

Arrange asparagus on a bed of shredded dark green lettuce. Combine chopped fruits, lemon juice, and sweetener if desired. Top each salad with one-fourth of the fruit mixture.

HEARTS OF ROMAINE

4 servings of
16 calories each

Ingredients

1 head romaine lettuce

Method

Quarter the head of romaine. Remove the coarse tips and place each heart on a chilled salad plate. Serve with favorite Spa dressing.

CUCUMBER VINAIGRETTE

4 servings of
16 calories each

Ingredients

1 large cucumber, unpeeled,
    sliced
2 oz. lemon juice
2 green onions, chopped fine
1 Tbsp. diced sweet red pepper
¼ cup white vinegar

½ cup unsweetened apple juice
dash white pepper
liquid sweetener to taste
    (optional)
pinch dry mustard

Method

Crisp the cucumber slices by packing in crushed ice. Drain. Combine remaining ingredients and marinate the cucumbers for 2–3 hours. Drain. Serve the cucumber slices on a bed of lettuce. No salad dressing its required.

ICEBERG LETTUCE MIMOSA

6 servings of
25 calories each

Ingredients

1 large head iceberg lettuce
½ cup julienned beets, no salt
    or sugar added

2 hard-cooked egg whites,
    chopped

Method

Cut the lettuce into six wedges. Crisp in crushed ice. Garnish the lettuce wedge with the julienned beets and chopped egg whites.

CELERY VINAIGRETTE

4 servings of
16 calories each

Ingredients

4 medium-size celery stalks
½ cup unsweetened apple juice
¼ cup white vinegar

1 Tbsp. fresh lemon juice
4 large lettuce cups

Method

Wash and cut the celery diagonally. Do not peel. Pour boiling water over the celery and drain at once. Combine apple juice, vinegar, and lemon juice; pour over the celery and marinate for 2–3 hours. Drain and serve in lettuce cups.

CAULIFLOWER VINAIGRETTE

6 servings of
16 calories each

Ingredients

1 medium head cauliflower
1 Tbsp. chopped sweet red
    pepper
½ cup unsweetened apple juice

¼ cup white vinegar
1 Tbsp. lemon juice
6 large lettuce cups

Method

Pour boiling water over the cauliflower and drain at once. Separate into flowerettes. Combine remaining ingredients and pour over the cauliflower; marinate for 2–3 hours. Serve in lettuce cups.

GREEN BEANS WITH SWEET RED PEPPERS, SCALLIONS, AND BOSTON LETTUCE

4 servings of
20 calories each

Ingredients

2 cups green beans, cooked
    without salt
4 scallions, cut very fine

1 Tbsp. diced sweet red pepper
Spa Vinaigrette Dressing
4 outer leaves of Boston lettuce

Method

Marinate the vegetables, except the Boston lettuce, in Spa Vinaigrette Dressing (page 182) for about 2 hours. Remove with a slotted spoon and arrange the salad on the lettuce leaves.

LA COSTA SPA SALAD

8 servings of
25 calories each

Ingredients

2 small green apples
2 cups shredded green cabbage
2 green peppers, seeded and
    sliced

1 Tbsp. lemon juice

Method

Core and chop the apples, leaving the skin on for color. Combine the apples, cabbage, green peppers, and lemon juice. Allow the salad to marinate for 2–3 hours before serving. Serve chilled on a lettuce leaf.

FRESH SPINACH SALAD

6 servings of
25 calories each

Ingredients

l lb. fresh spinach
2 hard-cooked egg whites,
    diced

l large tomato, cut into 6
    wedges

Method

Wash spinach thoroughly and remove any coarse stems. Place crisped spinach leaves in individual serving bowls. Top with diced egg whites and tomato wedges. Serve with favorite Spa dressing.

SLICED TOMATOES WITH FINES HERBES

4 servings of
16 calories each

Ingredients

2 small tomatoes, sliced
l Tbsp. chopped fresh parsley
l Tbsp. chopped chives

l Tbsp. chopped chervil
l Tbsp. chopped tarragon

Method

Arrange tomato slices attractively on individual salad plates. Sprinkle with the combined herbs. Serve with a Spa dressing.

HEARTS OF ROMAINE WITH RADISHES, ZUCCHINI, AND TOMATOES

4 servings of
16 calories each

Ingredients

l head romaine lettuce
4 red radishes, sliced
½ medium zucchini, sliced

l small tomato, cut into
    segments

Method

Cut the head of romaine into quarters. Cut off the tip of the core and crisp in crushed ice. Drain and garnish with radish slices, zucchini slices, and tomato segments. Serve with favorite Spa dressing.

COLESLAW

6 servings of
16 calories each

Ingredients

3 cups shredded green cabbage
1 small carrot, chopped
1 small green pepper, chopped
1 Tbsp. minced green onion
    tops

¼ cup unsweetened pineapple
    juice
¼ cup white vinegar

Method

Combine the vegetables. Pour the pineapple juice and vinegar over the mixture and marinate for 2 hours in refrigerator. Drain off the juice and serve the slaw well chilled.

ITALIAN SALAD BOWL

4 servings of
25 calories each

Ingredients

1 small head romaine, torn into
    bite-size pieces
1 zucchini, seeded and sliced
1 large tomato, cut into quarters

1 small red onion, sliced very
    thin and separated into
    rings
pinch oregano

Method

Chill romaine and zucchini in crushed ice. When crisp, fill small salad bowls and garnish with tomato and onion rings. Sprinkle with oregano. Serve with Spa Capri Dressing (page 183).

TOMATO PRINCESSE

4 servings of
16 calories each

Ingredients

3 small tomatoes, sliced

8 asparagus tips, cooked

Method

Arrange the tomato slices and asparagus on a bed of shredded lettuce. Serve with favorite Spa dressing.

MARINATED TOMATO SALAD

4 servings of
18 calories each

Ingredients

2 medium tomatoes, sliced thin
2 tsp. finely chopped onion

4 tsp. red wine vinegar
black pepper

Method

Arrange the tomato slices on individual plates and sprinkle onions, vinegar, and pepper on each. Refrigerate for 2 hours before serving.

≈≈≈≈≈≈≈≈≈≈≈≈≈≈≈≈≈≈≈≈≈≈≈≈≈

APPLE CELERY SALAD

6 servings of
25 calories each

Ingredients

1 large red delicious apple
juice of 1 lemon
4 stalks celery, washed and
    peeled

liquid artificial sweetener to
    taste

Method

Core and slice the apple (do not peel) and squeeze the fresh lemon juice over it (this keeps the apple from turning dark). Slice the celery diagonally in large pieces and mix with the apple slices. Add liquid sweetener and let the salad sit for one hour in the refrigerator. Arrange it in four portions on a bed of crisp lettuce and serve.

≈≈≈≈≈≈≈≈≈≈≈≈≈≈≈≈≈≈≈≈≈≈≈≈≈

APPLE CABBAGE SALAD

6 servings of
25 calories each

Ingredients

2 small golden delicious apples
1 Tbsp. lemon juice

2 cups shredded green cabbage
Spa Vinaigrette Dressing

Method

Wash, core, and slice the apples. Sprinkle with lemon juice. Combine the apples and cabbage and marinate in Spa Vinaigrette Dressing (page 182) for 1–2 hours in the refrigerator. Serve the drained salad on a leaf of lettuce.

CUCUMBER SLICES IN YOGURT WITH CHIVES

4 servings of
30 calories each

Ingredients

2 medium cucumbers,
    unpeeled
½ cup plain low-fat yogurt

3 Tbsp. chopped chives
pinch white pepper
small pinch dill

Method

Wash and slice the cucumbers about ¼ inch thick. Mix the yogurt with the remaining ingredients; add to the cucumber slices and marinate ½ hour. Serve well chilled.

BEAN SPROUTS, SCALLIONS, AND WATER CHESTNUTS

4 servings of
25 calories each

Ingredients

2 cups fresh bean sprouts,
    washed
4 green onion tops, chopped
    fine

8 water chestnuts, sliced
Spa Vinaigrette Dressing

Method

Combine the vegetables and marinate in the Spa Vinaigrette Dressing (page 182) for 20 minutes. Drain off the marinade and serve the salad chilled.

BOSTON LETTUCE AND AVOCADO

4 servings of
25 calories each

Ingredients

1 head Boston lettuce, cut into
    quarters

¼ avocado, sliced

Method

Wash and crisp the lettuce and place on serving plates. Arrange the avocado slices around the lettuce and serve with favorite Spa dressing.

CHIFFONADE SALAD

4 servings of
16 calories each

Ingredients

1 medium head purple cabbage
1 small carrot, shredded
2 stalks celery, peeled and
 sliced fine

1 Tbsp. shredded green pepper

Method

Wash and core cabbage. Shred and crisp in crushed ice. Drain. Toss the
vegetables and arrange on a salad plate. Serve with favorite Spa dressing.

PICKLED BEETS

4 servings of
36 calories each

Ingredients

2 cups canned beets, no salt or
 sugar added
1 Tbsp. red wine vinegar
1 bay leaf
1 whole clove

artificial sweetener to taste
 (optional)
½ small onion, sliced and
 separated into rings

Method

Drain the beet juice into a small skillet. Add the vinegar, bay leaf, clove, and
sweetener, bring to a boil, and simmer for one minute. Let the mixture cool.
Pour the cooled juice over the beets and allow to marinate overnight in the
refrigerator. Lift the beets from the juice with a slotted spoon and serve on a
bed of shredded lettuce. Garnish with the onion rings.

CITRUS BOUQUET SALAD

4 servings of
36 calories each

Ingredients

12 grapefruit sections
12 orange sections

crisp lettuce cups
4 Tbsp. Spa French Dressing

Method

Arrange grapefruit and orange sections alternately in the lettuce cups. Serve
with Spa French Dressing (page 183).

MARINATED CRISP FRESH VEGETABLES

4 servings of
36 calories each

Ingredients

8 fresh stalks asparagus
1 cup cauliflower buds
1 small carrot, sliced
½ small rutabaga, peeled and
   diced
1 zucchini, seeded and sliced

4 cherry tomatoes, cut in half
½ green pepper, seeded and
   sliced
½ cup unsweetened apple juice
¼ cup white vinegar
1 Tbsp. fresh lemon juice

Method

Cut the buds off the asparagus stalks and discard the stems. Scald the vegetables with boiling water and drain at once. Marinate the vegetables for 2–3 hours in the combined apple juice, vinegar, and lemon juice. Drain the vegetables and serve.

ORANGE GELATIN SALAD

6 servings of
40 calories each

Ingredients

2 medium carrots, peeled and
   shredded
1 orange, peeled and sectioned

1½ cups fresh orange juice
1½ cups water
1 Tbsp. plain gelatin

Method

Combine the shredded carrots, orange sections, and ¾ cup of the orange juice; set aside. Soften the gelatin in a little warm water and add the remaining orange juice and water. Combine the gelatin mixture with the carrot mixture, mixing well. Refrigerate the gelatin in a small baking pan until set. Cut into small squares and serve on a bed of shredded lettuce.

DRESSINGS

CUMBERLAND DRESSING

10 to 15 calories
per tablespoon

Ingredients

1 12-oz. bottle low-calorie
   ketchup (no sugar or
   salt added)
1 cup pure apple juice
juice of 1 lemon, strained
½ cup (4 oz.) red wine vinegar
1 tsp. dry mustard

1 cucumber, peeled
tops of 2 green onions
2 stalks celery hearts
1 green or red sweet pepper
Coarsely ground black pepper
Artificial sweetener to taste
   (optional)

Method

Blend all the ingredients except the vegetables, being careful to dissolve the mustard so there will be no lumps. Chop the vegetables fine and fold in just before serving to preserve freshness. Add black pepper and sweetener if desired.

SPA VINAIGRETTE DRESSING

10 calories
per tablespoon

Ingredients

¼ cup white vinegar
1 cup unsweetened pineapple
   juice
juice of ½ lemon, strained
¼ tsp. dry mustard
1 clove garlic, bruised

White pepper to taste
¼ cup each: finely chopped
   celery hearts, chives or
   green onion tops, green
   and red sweet peppers

Method

Blend well all ingredients except the chopped vegetables. (The garlic should be bruised only; it can then be removed before serving.) Add the chopped vegetables, place in a covered container, and refrigerate until served.

SPA CAPRI DRESSING
(Herbed Wine Vinegar)

10 calories
per tablespoon

Ingredients

2 cups red wine vinegar
pinch garlic powder
1 oz. chopped herbs to taste:
    basil
    oregano
    rosemary
    black pepper
    bay leaf

2 cups unsalted defatted beef
    broth, chilled
½ red onion, chopped very fine

Method

To the wine vinegar add the garlic powder and a wide variety of herbs and allow to stand overnight. Strain, and add chilled broth and onion.

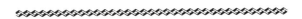

SPA FRENCH DRESSING

10 calories
per tablespoon

Ingredients

2 rounded tsp. vegetable gum
4 oz. (½ cup) white vinegar
12 oz. (1½ cups) unsweetened
    pineapple juice
juice of ½ lemon, strained

¼ level tsp. dry mustard
⅛ tsp. white pepper
3 heaping tsp. paprika
1 pinch ground celery seed

Method

Dissolve the vegetable gum in a small amount of the vinegar, or sprinkle the powdered gum very lightly on the top of the liquids, to prevent lumping. Mix the remainder of the vinegar, pineapple juice, lemon juice, mustard, pepper, paprika, and celery seed. Blend lightly with a wire whip or fork; do not overbeat. (If the dressing is overbeaten, the air incorporated dilutes the color.) Place in a covered container and store in the refrigerator until served.

There are many kinds of vegetable gum. They can be purchased from your pharmacist

SPA BUTTERMILK SALAD DRESSING

1 tablespoon per
serving;
10 calories
per tablespoon

Ingredients

1 cup unsalted tomato juice
1 cup red wine vinegar
1 tsp. dill weed
⅓ tsp. chervil

⅓ tsp. basil
1 tsp. oregano
pinch granulated garlic
1 pint buttermilk

Method

Combine the tomato juice, vinegar, and herbs and allow to marinate overnight.
Strain and add buttermilk. This will keep, refrigerated, for at least one week.

ENTREES

LA COSTA SPA SWEET AND SOUR SALMON

5 servings of
146 calories each

Ingredients

5 3-oz. salmon steaks
¼ cup red wine vinegar
1 cup water
1 shallot, chopped

1 Tbsp. pickling spice
1 tsp. cracked peppercorn
liquid artificial sweetener

Method

Combine all ingredients except salmon. Marinate salmon 2–3 hours in the mixture. In a shallow pan or skillet, heat the marinade to a simmer. Use a spatula to place the salmon steaks into the hot liquid. Cover lightly with foil. Cook salmon until it is opaque and flakes. Garnish each steak with 1 tablespoon poaching liquid.

BEEF CURRY

5 servings of
146 calories each

Ingredients

5 3-oz. lean beef tenderloins,
    from which all fat except
    the marbling has been
    removed (eye of
    tenderloin)
1 Tbsp. dry white wine
5 oz. (10 Tbsp.) unsweetened
    pineapple juice

pinch fresh chopped garlic
¼ tsp. curry powder
½ cup fresh pineapple cubes
    (¼")
1/3 cup plain shredded coconut
    (no sugar added), toasted
    slightly in the oven
pepper to taste

Method

Brown the beef fillets in a dry, very hot pan. Remove when medium rare. Use a spatula. Do not overload the pan. No juice will be lost by the meat if the pan is hot enough. To the brown meat glaze on the bottom of the pan, add the wine. Remove from the fire and allow the alcohol to evaporate. Do not burn the glaze. Add the remaining ingredients. The sauce should thicken in about 3 minutes. Replace the meat in the sauce to reheat. Remove each fillet to a hot plate, garnishing with the sauce to coat the meat and a few pineapple cubes on each fillet. Serve at once with a pinch of coconut on top.

SLICED BEEF PLATTER GARNI

4 servings of
146 calories each

Ingredients

6 oz. cold cooked New York
steak (lean only)
4 cups lettuce pieces

Spa Capri Dressing
½ cucumber, sliced
1 medium tomato, quartered

Method

Slice the steak crosswise, trimming off any excess fat. Marinate the lettuce in the Capri Dressing for a few minutes. Arrange the lettuce, cucumber, and tomato on individual serving plates. Top with the sliced steak. Serve with Spa Capri Dressing (page 183).

TUNA SALAD PLATE

4 servings of
146 calories each

Ingredients

2 3-oz. cans water-packed,
unsalted tuna
4 cups shredded lettuce

8 spears asparagus, cooked and
cooled
fresh parsley sprigs (optional)

Method

Drain the tuna and cut the contents of each can in half horizontally. Arrange on the shredded lettuce. Garnish with the asparagus spears and fresh parsley if desired.

BROILED MINUTE STEAK

4 servings of
146 calories each

Ingredients

4 3-oz. lean New York steak,
sliced thin

crushed black pepper

Method

Season the steaks with pepper and broil very quickly to desired doneness. Serve immediately.

COLD SOCKEYE SALMON PLATE

4 servings of
146 calories each

Ingredients

2 3-oz. cans water-packed
    unsalted sockeye salmon
4 cups shredded lettuce
8 cherry tomatoes

fresh parsley sprigs
1 small red onion, sliced and
    separated into rings

Method

Chill the salmon well before serving. Arrange the lettuce, cherry tomatoes, and parsley sprigs on individual serving platters. Slice the contents of each can of salmon in half horizontally. Place the chilled salmon in the center of each platter and top with the onion rings. Serve with favorite Spa dressing.

COLD LOBSTER PLATTER

1 serving of
146 calories each

Ingredients

3 oz. cold cooked lobster meat
2 stalks asparagus, cooked

2 diagonal slices raw carrot
1 cup shredded lettuce

Method

Arrange the lobster, asparagus, and carrot slices on top of the shredded lettuce. Serve with Spa Cocktail Sauce (page 222) and garnish with a lemon wedge if desired.

FRUIT PLATE WITH COTTAGE CHEESE

1 serving of
146 calories

Ingredients

2 oz. fresh pineapple, sliced
3 oz. fresh melon, sliced

3 oz. low-fat cottage cheese
dark salad greens

Method

Arrange the fruit on a bed of greens and place the cottage cheese in the center. Serve well chilled.

BEEF SHISH KABOB

4 servings of
146 calories each

Ingredients

10 oz. filet mignon, cut into 8
    cubes
½ cup dry red wine
½ cup water
1 Tbsp. chopped green onion
    tops

freshly ground pepper
pinch oregano
8 cherry tomatoes
8 fresh whole mushrooms
1 small green pepper, cut into
    8 squares

Method

Combine wine, water, onion tops, ground pepper, and oregano. Marinate the filet mignon cubes in this mixture for 1½ hours. Skewer filet mignon, tomatoes, mushrooms, and green pepper alternately on kabob sticks. Broil very quickly to desired doneness. Baste the kabobs with the marinade while broiling.

CHEF'S SALAD BOWL

1 serving of
146 calories

Ingredients

1 cup mixed salad greens
½ oz. unsalted cheddar cheese
½ oz. cooked chicken
½ oz. lean cooked beef
1 hard-cooked egg white,
    sliced

2 cherry tomatoes
2 spears cooked, cold
    asparagus

Method

Line a small salad bowl with a large lettuce cup. Fill with the mixed greens. Arrange the cheese, chicken, beef, egg white, cherry tomatoes, and cold asparagus on top of the greens. Serve with a Spa salad dressing.

PEPPER STEAK LA COSTA

4 servings of
146 calories each

Ingredients

4 3-oz. portions lean New
    York steak
½ cup unsalted defatted beef
    broth

2 thin slices onion
4 thin slices green pepper
4 mushrooms, sliced
black pepper

Method

Flatten the steaks lightly with a meat mallet. Place them in a hot nonstick frying pan or use a noncaloric vegetable spray. Brown the steaks quickly, turning once. Set aside. Deglaze the pan with the beef broth, stirring to loosen any particles of beef clinging to the pan. Add the remaining ingredients, stirring lightly. Cook only long enough for the vegetables to soften; they should still be crunchy. Garnish the top of each steak with a portion of the pepper sauce.

LAMB SHISH KABOB

4 servings of
146 calories each

Ingredients

10 oz. lean lamb, cut into
    8 cubes
½ cup dry burgundy
2 Tbsp. vinegar
4 Tbsp. water
2 Tbsp. chopped green onion
    tops

¼ tsp. garlic powder
¼ tsp. oregano
8 cherry tomatoes
8 fresh whole mushrooms
1 small green pepper, cut into
    8 squares

Method

Combine the wine, vinegar, water, onion tops, garlic powder, and oregano. Marinate the lamb in this mixture for 1½ hours. Skewer lamb, tomatoes, mushrooms, and green pepper alternately on kabob sticks. Broil very quickly under an open broiler or in a conventional oven-broiler. Brush the kabobs with the marinade while they cook.

ROAST SIRLOIN OF BEEF AU NATUREL

4 servings of
146 calories each

Ingredients

12 oz. New York steak, well
    trimmed

coarsely chopped fresh
    vegetables (onion, carrot,
    celery)

Method

Brown the meat in a very hot, dry skillet, then place it on a bed of coarsely chopped fresh vegetables. Roast at 475° to medium rare. The vegetables may be served as a garnish.

STUFFED BELL PEPPERS

4 servings of
146 calories each

Ingredients

4 small green peppers
½ pound lean ground beef
dash white pepper
1 cup unsalted whole tomatoes,
    chopped

¼ small yellow onion,
    chopped
¾ cup unsalted defatted beef
    broth

Method

Wash the green peppers and remove the seeds. Set aside. Brown the ground beef in a dry, hot pan and season with the pepper. Drain off all fat. Set aside. Combine one-half of the chopped tomatoes and all of the chopped onions. Simmer for a few minutes. Combine the ground beef and the tomato-onion mixture. Stuff each pepper with one-fourth of the ground beef mixture. Place the peppers in a shallow pan and pour the remaining chopped tomatoes and the beef broth around the peppers. Cover the pan with aluminum foil and bake for 45–60 minutes or until tender. Allow the peppers to cool slightly before serving. Reduce the liquid in the pan to one-half, and glaze each pepper with a little sauce.

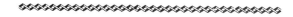

CHICKEN ALMANDINE

4 servings of
146 calories each

Ingredients

4 3½-oz. chicken breasts
½ cup unsweetened pineapple
    juice
½ cup unsalted, defatted
    chicken broth

pinch granulated garlic
white pepper to taste

Method

Remove all visible fat from the chicken. Brown in a hot (500°) oven for 15 minutes. Drain off all excess fat. As soon as the chicken has browned, reduce the oven to 325°. Combine the pineapple juice, chicken broth garlic, and white pepper and baste the chicken frequently while baking. Sprinkle the chicken pieces with the slivered almonds just before serving.

LINGUINI WITH CLAM SAUCE

4 servings of
200 calories each

Ingredients

1 medium shallot, minced
½ clove garlic, minced
1 medium tomato, peeled and
    diced
½ cup dietetic ketchup
juice from clams
4 oz. dietetic tomato juice

1 Tbsp. tomato paste
oregano
white pepper
½ cup clams, minced and
    drained
4 oz. linguini, uncooked
chopped fresh parsley

Method

Cook the linguini in boiling water until done. Drain. In a heavy skillet sauté the shallot and garlic in a little of the clam juice for 3 minutes. Combine the tomato, ketchup, juice, paste, and seasonings and stir. Simmer for half hour. Add the minced clams and heat through. Ladle the sauce over the cooked hot linguini and garnish with chopped parsley if desired.

LONDON BROIL WITH MUSHROOMS

4 serving of
146 calories each

Ingredients

4 3-oz. New York steaks, well
    trimmed
ground black pepper
½ cup unsalted, defatted beef
    broth

8 fresh mushrooms, sliced
1 shallot, chopped fine
1 tsp. chopped chives

Method

Season the steaks with the pepper. Place steaks in a hot, dry skillet which has been sprayed with a noncaloric vegetable spray. Cook the steaks quickly, turning once. Set aside. Deglaze the pan with the beef broth and stir in the mushrooms, shallot, and chives. Cook only long enough for the liquid to evaporate from the pan. Garnish each steak with the sautéed vegetables and serve.

COLD CHICKEN WITH FRUIT SALAD

4 servings of
146 calories each

Ingredients

6 oz. cold cooked chicken,
    sliced
shredded lettuce
1½ cups fresh melon cut into
    bite-size pieces
½ small orange, peeled and
    sectioned

½ cup fresh strawberries
¼ cup plain low-fat yogurt
2 Tbsp. orange juice
1 tsp. lime juice
artificial sweetener to taste
    (optional)

Method

Arrange the sliced chicken on a bed of shredded lettuce. Combine the melon, orange sections, and berries. Blend the yogurt, orange juice, and lime juice together (sweetener may be added here if desired). Combine the yogurt and fruit. Serve the chicken and fruit salad together on the same plate, or serve the fruit salad in separate dishes.

POACHED SALMON AMERICAINE

4 servings of
146 calories each

Ingredients

4 3-oz. salmon fillets, boned
2 Tbsp. dry white wine
1 Tbsp. lemon juice
1 cup water

1 Tbsp. diced carrot
1 Tbsp. diced onion
1 tomato, peeled and diced
2 oz. unsalted tomato juice

Method

Place the wine, lemon juice, and water in a heavy skillet and heat. Place the salmon fillets in the hot liquid and sprinkle the diced vegetables over the salmon. Cover and poach for approximately 10 minutes or until the fish is done. Remove the fish and keep it warm. Add the tomato juice to the stock and reduce the liquid by one-half. Ladle the sauce over the salmon and serve hot.

COQ AU VIN

4 servings of
146 calories each

Ingredients

4 3½-oz. chicken breasts
1 cup dry white wine
1 cup salt-free chicken broth
pinch thyme

white pepper
½ cup julienned carrots
½ cup sliced fresh mushrooms
½ cup pearl onions

Method

Brown the chicken in a 500° oven for 15 minutes; drain off all excess fat. Heat the wine and chicken broth in a heavy skillet; simmer for 10 minutes, uncovered. Pour the wine and chicken broth over the chicken; add the thyme, pepper, and carrots. Cover and cook until the chicken is done; remove chicken pieces. Add mushrooms and pearl onions; simmer the sauce and reduce by one-half. Glaze each chicken piece with some of the sauce.

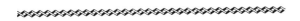

POACHED LOBSTER TAIL

4 servings of
146 calories each

Ingredients

4 5-oz. lobster tails in the shell
4 tsp. lemon juice

paprika
chopped parsley

Method

If frozen tails are used, thaw them. Take a heavy French knife and split the lobster shells lengthwise, deep enough to split the top shell layer and halfway through the lobster meat. Turn the shell over, lift out the lobster meat from the shell with your fingers, and squeeze the shell back together. Fold the lobster meat back over the closed shell. Repeat until each tail has been opened. Sprinkle the lobster meat with the lemon juice and paprika. Poach the tails in a heavy skillet with 2 inches of water. Only the shell should be covered with liquid. Cover lightly with foil and poach until the lobster meat is milky white; about 10 minutes — do not overcook. Garnish with chopped parsley.

CRAB MEAT NEW ORLEANS

4 servings of
146 calories each

Ingredients

12 oz. cooked crab meat
½ green pepper, cut into small
    pieces
1 medium tomato, peeled and
    diced
1 stalk celery, cut into small
    pieces

4 oz. unsalted tomato juice
1 oz. dietetic ketchup
white pepper
1 tsp. lemon juice

Method

Place all the ingredients except the crab meat into a saucepan and simmer until the vegetables are tender. Add the crab, and heat through. Serve at once in small casserole dishes.

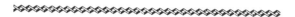

PAPRIKA CHICKEN

4 servings of
146 calories each

Ingredients

4 3½-oz. chicken breasts
white pepper
paprika
¼ cup dry white wine
¼ cup unsalted, defatted
    chicken broth

2 Tbsp. diced green pepper
½ tsp. finely chopped onion
pinch garlic powder
1 Tbsp. grated lemon rind
pinch caraway seeds

Method

Sprinkle the chicken breasts with white pepper and paprika; place in a shallow pan and bake uncovered at 375° for 30–40 minutes or until chicken is tender. Drain off all fat. Remove the chicken from the pan and set aside. Deglaze the pan with the white wine, allowing the alcohol to evaporate, then add the remaining ingredients. Reduce the sauce in the pan by one-half and ladle it over the chicken. Serve hot.

SALISBURY STEAK WITH MUSHROOMS

4 servings of
146 calories each

Ingredients

12 oz. lean chopped New York
   steak
½ cup unsalted, defatted beef
   broth

1 shallot, chopped fine
1 cup fresh sliced mushrooms

Method

Form four patties from the chopped meat; broil to desired doneness. Meanwhile, heat the beef broth in a heavy skillet and add the shallot and mushrooms. Simmer uncovered to reduce the sauce. Glaze each steak patty with a portion of the sauce. Serve very hot.

CURRY OF LAMB

4 servings of
146 calories each

Ingredients

4 3-oz. lamb chops, boned,
   with all the fat removed
Curry Sauce
1 small carrot, diced
1 stalk celery, diced
¼ cup shallots, peeled and
   finely chopped
½ cup diced unpeeled yellow
   apples

1 cup unsalted defatted chicken
   broth
½ cup unsweetened pineapple
   juice
1½ tsp. curry powder
pinch garlic powder
sprigs parsley, chopped fine

Method

Combine the vegetables and apple in a heavy saucepan; add the chicken broth and pineapple juice. Bring the mixture to a boil, then simmer slowly until reduced to one-half the original amount. Add the seasoning at the end of the cooking. Strain the sauce, using a wooden spoon to mash some of the vegetables through the strainer to thicken the sauce. Broil the lamb chops as desired; glaze each chop with the curry sauce. Garnish with parsley.

TENDERLOIN OF BEEF STROGANOFF

4 servings of
146 calories each

Ingredients

4 3-oz. strips tenderloin, with
    all fat trimmed off
2 tsp. dry burgundy
2 Tbsp. unsalted, defatted beef
    broth
2 large mushrooms, sliced

1 green onion, chopped
dash granulated garlic
black pepper to taste
2 heaping tsp. plain low-fat
    yogurt

Method

Heat a heavy skillet which has been sprayed with a noncaloric vegetable spray. Place the tenderloin strips in hot pan and brown, turning once. Remove the meat and keep it hot. Deglaze the pan with the burgundy, stirring to loosen any particles of beef clinging to the pan. Add the beef broth, mushrooms, green onions, and seasonings. Reduce the mixture until it becomes slightly thick. Add the yogurt, stirring only enough to combine. Do not let the mixture boil, as the yogurt will separate. Garnish each tenderloin with some of the sauce. Serve immediately.

HALIBUT JARDINIERE

4 servings of
146 calories each

Ingredients

4 3-oz. halibut fillets
¼ cup dry white wine
½ cup water
1 Tbsp. lemon juice

½ small onion, julienned
½ small carrot, julienned
1 small stalk celery, julienned
white pepper (optional)

Method

Combine the wine, water, and lemon juice in a skillet. Bring to a light boil. Place the halibut in the hot liquid. Sprinkle julienned vegetables over the top of each fillet; cover and simmer gently for approximately 10 minutes. Remove the fillets to a hot serving platter, leaving the vegetables in the skillet. Reduce the sauce by one-half and spoon the vegetables and sauce over the fillets. Sprinkle with a little white pepper if desired. Serve at once.

BROILED TROUT WITH FRESH DILL

4 servings of
146 calories each

Ingredients

2 8-oz. frozen or fresh trout
white pepper

1 Tbsp. lemon juice
chopped fresh dill

Method

Bone the trout and slice each in half to make four fillets. Sprinkle the fillets with white pepper and lemon juice. Place the fillets on the rack of a broiler pan which has been sprayed with a noncaloric vegetable spray; or fill the bottom of the broiler pan with chopped raw vegetables (this prevents the delicate fish from drying out). Broil for six to seven minutes or until done.

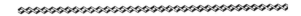

POACHED FLOUNDER

4 servings of
146 calories each

Ingredients

4 3-oz. fresh or frozen flounder
    fillets
2 cups water
1 shallot, peeled and chopped
3 sprigs parsley
1 small stalk celery, sliced

1 small yellow onion
1 bay leaf
1 whole clove
1 paprika
4 slices lemon

Method

If using frozen fish, thaw and retain any juice that leaks from the fish. Combine fish juice, 2 cups water, shallot, parsley, and celery. Peel the onion and stick the clove, together with the bay leaf, into the onion. Add to the fish broth. Cover the broth and simmer for 10 minutes. Strain. Ladle the broth into a heavy skillet and gently place the fish fillets in the liquid. Cover the skillet lightly with aluminum foil and poach gently approximately 10 minutes or until the fish is just tender. Serve with paprika and a slice of lemon for garnish.

ROAST LEG OF LAMB WITH MINT SAUCE

146 calories per
serving
(with mint sauce)

Ingredients

Mint Sauce
⅓ cup unsweetened apple
   juice
⅓ cup unsweetened pineapple
   juice

1 Tbsp. red wine vinegar
Fresh mint leaves, chopped
   fine

Method

Take one whole leg of lamb and trim off all visible fat. Season with a little white pepper, garlic powder, and rosemary. Roast at 400° F until medium rare, then allow to rest, so that by serving time it should be medium. Serve 2 ounces of thin-sliced lamb per person.

Combine liquids and chopped mint leaves; heat through. Add artificial sweetener if necessary. Serve on the side in small dip cups.

SCAMPI

4 servings of
146 calories each

Ingredients

16 oz. (1 lb.) medium-sized
   raw, shelled shrimp
2 medium tomatoes, peeled
   and diced
1 tsp. finely chopped shallots

¼ cup chopped green pepper
white pepper to taste
lemon juice
1 Tbsp. white wine
½ clove garlic, minced

Method

Devein and wash shrimp. Spray a heavy skillet with a noncaloric vegetable spray and heat. Place the shrimp in the skillet and pan-broil very quickly. When they are done and a little brown, remove them from the skillet. Place the diced tomato, shallots, and green pepper in the skillet. Season with pepper, lemon juice, wine, and garlic. Toss gently. Bring the mixture to a simmer and put the scampi back into the vegetable mixture to reheat. Serve in a small casserole.

COBB SALAD BOWL

1 serving of
200 calories

Ingredients

¼ head iceberg lettuce
¼ head romaine lettuce
½ bunch fresh watercress
a few leaves of endive
½ oz. unsalted cheddar cheese,
   diced
½ oz. cooked chicken meat,
   diced

½ oz. cooked roast beef, diced
½ tomato, peeled and diced
⅛ avocado, peeled and sliced
1 hard-cooked egg white,
   chopped

Method

Chop the lettuces, watercress, and endive together until fine and well mixed. Line a large individual salad bowl with a leaf of lettuce, and fill with the chopped greens. Arrange the remaining ingredients in the salad bowl and serve with a Spa salad dressing.

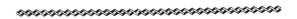

BROILED SOLE WITH CURRIED HORSERADISH SAUCE

4 servings of
146 calories each

Ingredients

4 3-oz. sole fillets, boned
1 Tbsp. lemon juice
white pepper
1 Tbsp. dry white wine

½ cup plain low-fat yogurt
2 tsp. grated horseradish
curry powder to taste

Method

Sprinkle the fillets with lemon juice and white pepper. Place the wine in the bottom of a nonstick pan and then add the fish fillets. Broil quickly, about 4–5 minutes. Do not turn the fillets. Combine the sauce ingredients and serve on the side. Garnish the sole with lemon slices and parsley if desired.

CHICKEN CACCIATORE

4 servings of
146 calories each

Ingredients

4 3½-oz. chicken breasts
4 medium-size tomatoes,
   peeled and chopped
1 slice onion

pinch each oregano, rosemary,
   and basil
1 clove garlic, minced
½ 4-oz. bottle dietetic ketchup

Method

Trim the chicken of all excess fat. Brown in a hot oven (500°F) for 15 minutes. Combine remaining ingredients and pour over the chicken. Return the chicken to the oven and bake at 350°, covered, for 30 minutes.

TOSTADA

4 servings of
200 calories each

Ingredients

4 small cornmeal tortilla shells
6 oz. lean ground meat
white pepper
1 tsp. chili powder
1 Tbsp. chopped onion
1 medium tomato, chopped
¼ head lettuce, shredded

½ oz. salt-free cheddar cheese,
   shredded
Hot Sauce
1 medium tomato, chopped
1 Tbsp. chopped onion
2 green onions, chopped
1 whole yellow chili pepper

Method

Combine the sauce ingredients; chill well. Crisp the tortilla shells in the oven at 350° for about 10 minutes; set aside. Sauté the ground meat in a heavy skillet, drain off all fat, and season with pepper and chili powder. Place one-fourth of the meat mixture on each tortilla shell and top with the remaining ingredients. Place the completed tostada under the broiler for 30 seconds to melt the cheese. Serve with the sauce.

SPA SWISS STEAK

4 servings of
146 calories each

Ingredients

4 3-oz. New York steaks
white pepper to taste
garlic powder to taste
¼ cup diced onion

½ cup diced fresh tomato
½ cup unsalted, defatted beef
   broth
½ cup unsalted tomato juice

Method

Season the steaks with the pepper and garlic; brown in a hot skillet which has been sprayed with a noncaloric vegetable spray. When brown, remove the meat and add the onion to the pan, sautéing until brown. Add the diced tomatoes, beef broth, and tomato juice. Place the steaks into the sauce and braise them covered, in a 375° oven until tender. Remove the meat ahead of time and reduce the sauce to one-half. Ladle the sauce over the steaks before serving.

LOBSTER AMBASSADOR

4 servings of
146 calories each

Ingredients

12 oz. cooked lobster meat
½ green pepper, cut into small
    pieces
1 medium tomato, peeled and
    diced
1 stalk celery, cut into small
    pieces

4 oz. dietetic tomato juice
1 oz. dietetic ketchup
white pepper to taste
2 tsp. lemon juice

Method

Place all ingredients except the lobster meat in a saucepan and simmer until tender. Then add the lobster meat and heat through. Serve hot.

MEDALLION OF VEAL PRINCESS

4 servings of
146 calories each

Ingredients

12 oz. trimmed veal, cut into 4
    steaks
1/3 cup dry white wine
1 cup fresh mushrooms, sliced

8 canned asparagus spears
    (dietetic pack)
white pepper
chopped parsley

Method

Pound the veal lightly with a meat mallet to flatten. Heat a heavy skillet which has been sprayed with a noncaloric vegetable spray and brown the veal on both sides. Remove veal and set aside. Deglaze the pan with the wine. Add the mushrooms and sauté. Cut the tips off the asparagus spears and discard the stems. Add the asparagus tips, pepper, and parsley to the sautéed mushrooms and heat through. Return the veal to the vegetable mixture and simmer for 5 minutes. Serve hot.

FLUFFY CREOLE OMELETTE

4 servings of
146 calories each

Ingredients

Omelette
8 eggs
salt substitute, to taste
white pepper to taste
Creole Sauce
¼ small yellow onion, sliced

½ whole green pepper, seeded
    and sliced
½ small tomato, peeled and
    diced
1 Tbsp. dietetic ketchup

Method

To make sauce: Heat a heavy skillet which has been sprayed with a noncaloric vegetable spray, and sauté the sliced onion until done but not brown. Add the pepper, tomato, and ketchup. Simmer until the vegetables are done, approximately 10–15 minutes.

Make one omelette at a time. Beat two eggs until frothy, adding a pinch of salt substitute, white pepper, and ½ teaspoon water. Cook the omelette in a hot nonstick pan over low heat until the bottom is set and slightly brown. Place about one-fourth of the Creole Sauce in the center of the omelette, fold the omelette in half, and slide it onto a plate. Repeat until all four omelettes are made.

HALIBUT IN WINE SAUCE

4 servings of
146 calories each

Ingredients

4 3-oz. halibut fillets
½ cup white wine or Spa Court
    Bouillon (p. 124)
½ cup unsalted, defatted fish
    broth
1 shallot, chopped fine

2 sprigs parsley, chopped
1 tsp. arrowroot
1/3 cup nonfat milk
white pepper
1 tsp. lemon juice

Method

Combine the wine, fish broth, chopped shallot, and parsley in a heavy skillet. (If fish broth is not available, substitute water.) Heat to boiling, and then simmer 5–10 minutes, covered. Place the halibut in the hot liquid and poach gently about 10 minutes. Remove the fillets and keep warm. Dilute the arrowroot in the nonfat milk. Combine it slowly with the hot fish broth, stirring constantly until the sauce is the consistency of a thin gravy. Season it with the white pepper and lemon juice. Return the halibut to the sauce and simmer for 2 minutes.

ROAST DUCK

4 servings of
146 calories each

Ingredients

1 2-lb. duck
white pepper
6 carrots, sliced

3 onions, sliced
8 stalks celery, sliced

Method

Wash the duck and remove the neck, gizzard, and giblets. Sprinkle the cavity with a little pepper. Stuff the cavity with about 1/3 of the vegetables. Tie the legs together so the vegetables won't fall out. To remove much of the duck fat, place the whole duck in a large pot with 2 quarts of boiling water, and boil for 10 minutes. Remove the duck and pat it dry with a clean napkin or paper towel. Squeeze the duck during this process, as more and more fat will be extracted.

Place the remaining chopped vegetables on the bottom of a large roasting pan and place the duck on top of the vegetables. This adds moistness to the duck and prevents the duck from sitting in any fat residue while roasting. Roast the duck at 425° until it begins to turn brown, approximately 20 minutes. Do not baste and do not turn the duck at any time during the cooking. Once the duck browns, reduce the oven temperature to 350°. The entire roasting time should take only about 2–2½ hours.

The duck is ready when the skin is crisp and the leg meat feels tender to touch. Remove the duck from the roasting pan and slice in half lengthwise; discard all the vegetables inside. Peel off the breast and hip bones. Place the duck pieces on bread slices skin side up and place under the broiler for a few minutes to crisp. Much excess fat is absorbed by the bread slices this way. (Discard the bread before serving.) Serve the duck accompanied by hot unsweetened applesauce if desired.

BROILED SALMON STEAKS

4 servings of
146 calories each

Ingredients

4 3-oz. salmon fillets
4 tsp. lemon juice

white pepper (optional)
4 lemon slices

Method

Season salmon fillets with the lemon juice and a little white pepper if desired. Broil until well done but not dry. Garnish each fillet with chopped parsley and serve with a lemon slice if desired.

VEAL CUTLETS

4 servings of
146 calories each

Ingredients

12 oz. trimmed veal, cut into 4
    steaks
1/3 cup dry white wine
8 fresh mushrooms, sliced
1 medium tomato, peeled and
    chopped

1 scallion, chopped fine
white pepper
garlic powder

Method

Flatten the veal steaks with a meat mallet. Heat a heavy skillet which has been sprayed with a noncaloric vegetable spray. Brown the veal in the skillet; remove and keep warm. Deglaze the skillet with the wine and stir to loosen any particles on the bottom of the pan. Add the mushrooms, tomato, scallion, and seasonings. Simmer about 5 minutes, then add the veal cutlets. Simmer 2 minutes longer.

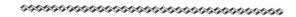

CHICKEN IN THE POT WITH NOODLES

4 servings of
200 calories each

Ingredients

1 2-lb. whole chicken
white pepper
1 bay leaf
½ cup diced carrot

1 celery stalk, cut into ½-in.
    pieces
1 rutabaga, peeled and diced
2 oz. thin noodles (raw weight)

Method

Place the chicken in a large pot and cover with cold water. Add all remaining ingredients except noodles. Bring to a boil and simmer covered for 2–2½ hours. Remove the vegetables from the stock with a slotted spoon as soon as they are done and set aside. When the chicken is cooked, remove it. Strain the stock and return it to the skillet. Add the noodles and simmer until they are tender. Replace the vegetables into the stock and cut the chicken into pieces; place the chicken pieces into large soup bowls and ladle the stock over the chicken. Serve very hot.

TROUT CAPRI

4 servings of
200 calories each

Ingredients

2 6-oz. trout, boned and cut in
    half lengthwise
white pepper
1 Tbsp. fresh lemon juice
1 Tbsp. dry white wine

2 Tbsp. fresh orange juice
¼ cup unsalted chicken broth
1 tsp. chopped shallots
½ banana, sliced thin
8 orange slices

Method

Place the trout fillets skin side down in a shallow pan. Sprinkle with pepper and lemon juice; moisten with the wine, orange juice, and chicken broth. Add the shallots. Poach the trout until tender, about 4–5 minutes. Remove to serving plates and keep warm. Place banana slices and two orange slices on top of each fillet. Reduce remaining poaching stock to one-half, then pour a little over each fillet and serve very hot. Garnish each with a sprig of parsley and a lemon wedge if desired.

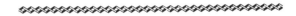

SPRING CHICKEN WITH LEMON AND GINGER

4 servings of
146 calories each

Ingredients

4 3½-oz. chicken breasts
1 cup unsalted, defatted
    chicken broth
1 Tbsp. lemon juice

pinch garlic powder
freshly grated ginger
white pepper to taste

Method

Remove all visible fat from the chicken. Brown in a 500° oven for 15 minutes. Drain off all fat. Combine chicken broth, lemon juice, garlic, and white pepper in a heavy skillet. Add enough fresh ginger to suit your taste. Simmer the broth uncovered until it is reduced by one-half. Reduce the oven temperature to 350° and bake the chicken uncovered about 30 minutes. Baste the chicken frequently while baking with the lemon-ginger sauce.

BROILED FILET MIGNON

4 servings of
146 calories each

Ingredients

4 3-oz. filet mignon steaks   white pepper

Method

Remove all fat from the steaks. Sprinkle with pepper and broil to desired doneness.

VEGETABLES

BROILED EGGPLANT PARMESAN

4 servings of
40 calories each

Ingredients

1 medium eggplant
2 Tbsp. grated Parmesan cheese

white pepper

Method

Wash the eggplant well and cut off both ends. Slice the eggplant into four round slices, about one-half inch thick. Sprinkle each with a little white pepper and the cheese. Place the slices on a baking sheet and bake uncovered in a 400° oven for 10–12 minutes or until tender.

❈❈❈❈❈❈❈❈❈❈❈❈❈❈❈❈❈❈❈❈❈❈❈

LA COSTA SPA SPINACH IN RED WINE

4½-cup servings
of 20 calories each

Ingredients

¼ cup chicken or beef broth
1 cup fresh mushrooms, sliced
1 clove garlic, pressed
¼ tsp. dry mustard
¼ cup dry red wine

1 10-oz. package frozen
    spinach or 1 lb. fresh (2
    cups cooked and drained)
salt substitute to taste
pepper to taste

Method

Heat the broth in a large heavy pan or skillet. Add the mushrooms, clove of garlic, and dry mustard; simmer for 5 minutes. Discard the garlic. Add the wine while the pan is very hot; this allows the alcohol to evaporate. Add the spinach and season to taste. Keep covered until time to serve.

Vegetables should be served very hot or very cold, never lukewarm.

CELERY JULIENNE WITH SWEET RED PEPPER

4 servings of
16 calories each

Ingredients

6 tender stalks celery, cut into
    small strips
1 Tbsp. chopped sweet red
    pepper

white pepper

Method

Drop the celery into boiling water and simmer, covered, until tender. Drain well and toss with the red pepper. Sprinkle with white pepper. Serve hot.

    Note: The peppers used here are the same as those which are marinated in oil and called pimientos. They can be purchased water-packed.

BROILED EGGPLANT SLICES

4 servings of
16 calories each

Ingredients

1 medium eggplant, peeled

white pepper

Method

Slice the eggplant into ½-inch-thick round slices. Season with white pepper and broil for about 5 to 8 minutes.

JULIENNE OF RUTABAGA

4 servings of
35 calories each

Ingredients

2 cups peeled, julienned
    rutabaga

chopped parsley

Method

Boil the julienned rutabaga in water until fork-tender. Drain and toss with chopped parsley.

PARSLEYED CAULIFLOWER

6 servings of
16 calories each

Ingredients

1 medium head cauliflower
fresh chopped parsley

paprika (optional)

Method

Wash, core, and break the cauliflower into small flowerettes. Drop into boiling water and simmer until tender — do not overcook. Remove with a slotted spoon. Toss with a little fresh parsley and paprika if desired.

CHOPPED SPINACH

6 servings of
16 calories each

Ingredients

1 lb. fresh spinach leaves

2 Tbsp. fresh lemon juice

Method

Wash the spinach leaves well and discard the stems. Simmer in boiling water, covered, until fork tender. Drain the spinach and season with the lemon juice. Toss gently. Serve at once.

HUNGARIAN BRUSSELS SPROUTS

4 servings of
16 calories each

Ingredients

2 cups Brussels sprouts
¼ small fresh tomato, peeled
    and diced

paprika

Method

Boil the Brussels sprouts in water to cover until fork-tender. Drain and toss with the diced tomato. Sprinkle with paprika before serving.

LA COSTA SPA RATATOUILLE

5 servings of
16 calories each

Ingredients

½ small red onion, sliced thin
1 clove garlic, minced
½ small green pepper, sliced
1 16-oz. can whole tomatoes
1 cup zucchini chunks
1 cup peeled and cubed
    eggplant

1½ tsp. oregano
1½ tsp. chopped parsley
black pepper
salt substitute and artificial
    sweetener to taste

Method

In a heavy saucepan, mix the sliced onion, minced garlic, sliced green pepper, and tomatoes cut into bite-size pieces. To prepare the zucchini, split into fourths lengthwise. Remove the seeds and soft center, and cut into bite-size pieces. To prepare the eggplant, peel and cut into ½-inch cubes. Add oregano, chopped parsley, and pepper. Toss together. Bring the mixture to the boiling point, reduce the heat to simmer, and cook until fork-tender. Adjust the seasoning as desired. This dish is better when held and reheated.

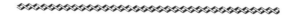

AVOCADO ON THE HALF SHELL WITH SHRIMP SALAD

2 servings of
200 calories each

Ingredients

1 oz. cooked shrimp
4 Tbsp. whipped low-fat
    cottage cheese
2 Tbsp. diced celery hearts
pinch chives

⅛ tsp. dry mustard
white pepper to taste
1 small avocado, about 6 in.
    long

Method

Combine shrimp, whipped cottage cheese, celery, chives, dry mustard, and white pepper. Peel and split the avocado in half, removing the pit. Stuff each avocado half with one-half the shrimp salad. Serve on a bed of dark greens with lemon wedges. (Do not let the peeled avocado stand for a long time; it will turn dark.)

FRENCH PEAS

4 servings of
36 calories each

Ingredients

2 cups fresh green peas
liquid artificial sweetener to
    taste

¼ cup shredded lettuce
8 pearl onions, unsalted

Method

Boil the peas until tender in water with a little sweetener. When the peas are cooked, drain off most of the water. Add the lettuce and pearl onions; heat only enough to wilt the lettuce and heat the onions. Drain and serve.

ASPARAGUS SPEARS

4 servings of
16 calories each

Ingredients

12 fresh asparagus spears
white pepper

1 bay leaf

Method

Add all ingredients to 2 cups boiling water. Cook until the asparagus is tender.

FRESH BROCCOLI WITH LEMON

4 servings of
16 calories each

Ingredients

1 lb. fresh broccoli, trimmed
2 lemon slices

1 lemon to garnish

Method

Cut the broccoli into small stalks. Add the lemon slices to 2 cups boiling water. Add the broccoli and simmer, covered, until tender. Garnish the broccoli with thin lemon slices or serve with lemon wedges.

BABY CARROTS À L'ORANGE

4 servings of
36 calories each

Ingredients

2 large carrots, peeled and
sliced
1½ cups unsalted chicken
broth

1 medium green onion,
chopped
1 small orange, peeled and
diced

Method

Heat the chicken broth to boiling. Add the carrots and green onion; cover and cook until nearly tender, approximately 7–8 minutes. Add the diced orange and cook 4–5 minutes more. Serve hot.

HOT SPICED BEETS

4 servings of
36 calories each

Ingredients

2 cups dietetic canned beets,
sliced
2 cloves
1 bay leaf

1 Tbsp. red wine vinegar
liquid sweetener to taste
(optional)

Method

Drain the juice from the beets. Bring the juice to a boil with the cloves and bay leaf. Add the vinegar and sweetener. Heat 10 minutes. Remove the cloves and bay leaf. Add the beets to the hot liquid and heat through for approximately one minute. Serve hot.

MUSHROOMS WITH CHERRY TOMATOES

4 servings of
16 calories each

Ingredients

16 medium-size fresh
mushrooms
12 cherry tomatoes

⅓ cup unsalted, defatted
chicken broth
chopped parsley

Method

Wash and quarter the mushrooms. Wash and slice the cherry tomatoes in half. Heat the chicken broth in a skillet and add the mushrooms. When the mushrooms are partially cooked, add the cherry tomatoes and simmer for one minute. Drain the vegetables and serve hot. Garnish with a little chopped parsley.

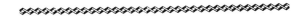

DICED ZUCCHINI SQUASH

4 servings of
16 calories each

Ingredients

2 medium zucchini
white pepper
½ tsp. chopped parsley
½ tsp. chives

1 tsp. chopped green onion
    tops
1 Tbsp. chopped celery leaves

Method

Wash and dice the zucchini into bite-size pieces. Sprinkle the remaining ingredients over the zucchini; toss gently. Bake in a covered shallow pan at 350° for 30 minutes.

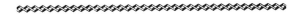

DICED CELERY AND CARROTS

4 servings of
26 calories each

Ingredients

2 medium carrots, peeled and
    sliced
3 stalks celery, sliced
    diagonally

chopped parsley

Method

Cook the vegetables separately in a small amount of boiling water (celery takes longer to cook than carrots). Combine the vegetables just before serving. Toss with fresh chopped parsley.

GREEN BEANS WITH SCALLIONS

4 servings of
16 calories each

Ingredients

½ lb. fresh green beans
2 medium scallions, chopped
    fine

Method

Wash beans and remove strings. Cut beans as desired. Bring one cup of water to a boil. Drop the green beans into the boiling water and cook until tender. Drain the beans and place in a hot serving dish; sprinkle with the scallions and toss gently.

GREEN BEANS ITALIENNE

4 servings of
16 calories each

Ingredients

1½ cups fresh green beans
dash pepper
dash garlic powder

1 small tomato, peeled and
    diced

Method

Wash beans and remove strings; cut in half horizontally. Boil them in a small amount of water seasoned with pepper and garlic. When green beans are barely tender drain them. Combine the green beans with the tomato and braise slowly for 3 minutes. Serve very hot.

PEAS AND CARROTS

4 servings of
36 calories each

Ingredients

⅓ cup unsalted chicken broth
1 cup fresh green peas

1 cup diced fresh carrots

Method

Heat the chicken broth to the boiling point and add the peas and carrots. Simmer covered for 3–4 minutes or until fork-tender. Take the vegetables out with a slotted spoon and serve hot.

BAKED TOMATOES PARMESAN

4 servings of
25 calories each

Ingredients

4 small tomatoes (2–2½ in. diameter)

3 tsp. grated Parmesan cheese

Method

Make a crossed incision on the top of each tomato and remove the core. Drop the tomatoes in hot water for one minute or until the skin can be easily removed. Set the peeled tomatoes in a shallow pan and sprinkle each with Parmesan cheese. Bake in a 350° oven for 10 minutes. Serve hot.

BEAN SPROUTS WITH MUSHROOMS

4 servings of
16 calories each

Ingredients

½ cup unsalted chicken broth
1 cup fresh bean sprouts

½ cup sliced fresh mushrooms

Method

Heat the chicken broth and add the bean sprouts and mushrooms. Simmer for 5 minutes only. Drain the vegetables and serve hot.

MIXED FRESH VEGETABLES

4 servings of
36 calories each

Ingredients

½ cup sliced carrots
½ cup cut green beans
4 cauliflower buds
¼ cup diced rutabaga

1 bay leaf
1 medium tomato, peeled and diced

Method

Combine all ingredients except tomato with one quart of boiling water. Simmer covered for 5 minutes. Add the diced tomato, drain the vegetables and serve hot. Garnish with chopped parsley if desired.

WHIPPED SQUASH

4 servings of
36 calories each

Ingredients

1 12-oz. package frozen
   whipped winter squash
1 Tbsp. unsweetened apple
   juice

ground cinnamon (optional)

Method

Combine the thawed squash, apple juice, and cinnamon if desired; blend
thoroughly. Heat the squash and serve hot.

FRESH ARTICHOKES WITH HOT DIP

4 servings of
36 calories each

Ingredients

4 small artichokes
4 thick slices lemon
Dip
1 cup salt-free chicken broth

1 tsp. lemon juice
½ tsp. chopped parsley
½ tsp. dill

Method

Wash the artichokes and cut off the tips (or thorns) of each leaf. Place each
artichoke on a slice of lemon in a large shallow skillet. Add enough boiling
water to half fill the skillet. Cover and cook until tender, about 12 minutes.
Take the skillet off the heat and allow the artichokes to steep for 2 to 3 minutes.
To make dip, combine cold broth, lemon juice, dill and garnish with parsley.
Heat and serve.

SAVORY GREEN BEANS

4 servings of
16 calories each

Ingredients

2 cups fresh green beans
2 tsp. chives
1 Tbsp. finely chopped green
   onion tops

1 sprig fresh parsley, chopped
white pepper

Method

Wash and cut the green beans lengthwise. Cook in boiling water until tender. Drain well. Toss the beans with the remaining ingredients and serve.

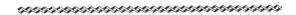

SWEET AND SOUR RED CABBAGE

4 servings of
16 calories each

Ingredients

2 cups shredded red cabbage
½ cup chicken stock
1 green onion top, chopped
    fine

⅓ cup red wine vinegar
¼ cup unsweetened apple juice
1 bay leaf
2 whole cloves

Method

Combine stock, green onion top, vinegar, apple juice, bay leaf, and cloves. Bring to a boil. Add the cabbage and simmer covered for about 30 minutes.

    The secret to a good sweet and sour cabbage is to cook it long enough so that the liquid has evaporated and the cabbage retains its beautiful color.

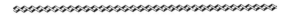

TOASTED POTATO SHELLS

4 servings of
30 calories each

Ingredients

2 medium baking potatoes
1 Tbsp. chopped chives

1 tsp. Parmesan cheese
½ tsp. caraway seeds

Method

Wash and bake the potatoes in a hot oven (500°) for 45 minutes to one hour or until done. The skins should be a little crisp. Cut the potatoes in half while hot, and scoop out the potato flesh (which can be served mashed the following day) leaving ⅓ inch nearest the skin. Place the shells back in the oven at 350° for 10 minutes or until fairly crisp. Combine the chives, Parmesan cheese, and caraway seeds; sprinkle a little in each shell and return to the oven just long enough for the cheese to melt.

YELLOW CROOKNECK SQUASH WITH FRENCH PEAS

4 servings of
25 calories each

Ingredients

1 cup sliced yellow crookneck
   squash (washed and
   seeded)

1 cup unsalted chicken broth
1 cup frozen peas

Method

Bring the broth to a boil and add the crookneck squash. Cover and allow to simmer for 5 minutes. Add the peas and cook for 5 minutes longer. Drain the vegetables and serve. Garnish with chopped parsley

BAKED HUBBARD SQUASH

4 servings of
36 calories each

Ingredients

1 small hubbard squash
   (approx. 1 lb.)
½ cup orange juice

ground cinnamon
nutmeg

Method

Cut the squash into four pieces and remove the seeds. Braise the squash, covered, in a shallow pan until somewhat softened, about 10 to 15 minutes. Sprinkle with orange juice, cinnamon, and nutmeg. Bake the squash in the oven uncovered at 350° for about 20 to 25 minutes or until a fork can pierce the squash easily.

CRISP CHINESE PEA PODS

6 servings of
16 calories each

Ingredients

1 lb. Chinese (snow) pea pods

Method

Steam the pea pods in one cup water for 2–3 minutes only. The pea pods should be crisp when served. A few drops of lemon juice will hold the bright green color. Serve immediately.

ZUCCHINI PROVENÇALE

4 servings of
16 calories each

Ingredients

2 medium zucchini
1 shallot, peeled
1 small tomato, peeled and
    diced

pinch granulated garlic

Method

Wash and slice the zucchini about ⅓ inch thick. Heat a heavy skillet which has been sprayed with a noncaloric vegetable spray. Sauté the shallot and tomato covered. Season with the garlic. When some liquid from the tomato has coated the bottom of the pan, add the zucchini and simmer covered for 3 minutes or until tender. Toss lightly and serve. Do not overcook.

BRAISED LETTUCE

4 servings of
16 calories each

Ingredients

½ head of romaine lettuce
½ cup unsalted chicken broth
½ cup julienned carrots

1 shallot, peeled
white pepper

Method

Wash the romaine and remove some of the outer leaves and the core. Tear the lettuce into bite-size pieces. Heat the chicken broth to boiling, and add the carrots and shallot. Simmer for 3 minutes, covered. Add the lettuce and a dash of white pepper. Cover and braise approximately 10 minutes. Remove the vegetables with a slotted spoon. Serve hot.

BAKED RED ONIONS

4 servings of
36 calories each

Ingredients

1 large red onion, peeled and sliced

Method

Place the onion slices on foil-covered baking pan in a hot oven (400°). Brown the onions on both sides. Serve hot.

HOT CABBAGE WEDGES

4 servings of
16 calories each

Ingredients

1 small head green cabbage
1 cup unsalted chicken broth

chopped parsley

Method

Wash and remove the outer leaves of the cabbage; core and cut the cabbage into four wedges. Place the cabbage wedges in a baking pan and pour the chicken broth over the wedges. Cover and bake at 350° for 20 minutes or until the cabbage is tender. Garnish each wedge with a little chopped parsley.

CABBAGE WITH SWEET PEPPERS

4 servings of
20 calories each

Ingredients

2 cups shredded green cabbage
1 green pepper, shredded
½ cup unsweetened apple
   juice

½ small onion, sliced
1 tsp. white vinegar
white pepper

Method

Combine the shredded green cabbage and green pepper. In a heavy skillet, heat the apple juice to the boiling point. Add the onion, vinegar, and finally the cabbage and peppers. Sprinkle with white pepper and braise, covered, for about 15 minutes or until tender. Remove with a slotted spoon and serve very hot.

FILLERS

MEAT GLAZE

Method

Meat glaze is made by professional chefs by browning veal bones and meat in a very hot oven. Do not use meat concentrates. Transfer to a pot, cover with a bouquet of vegetables and cold water. Cook slowly 6–8 hours, strain, clarify with egg white and strain again. Reduce to a rich brown sauce. Refrigerate and use as a base for Spa sauces. Use sparingly, as calorie count is difficult to estimate.

JAM

10 calories
per teaspoon

Ingredients

1 quart unsweetened fruit
lemon juice to taste
1 tsp. plain gelatin, dissolved
    in a little water

liquid artificial sweetener to
taste

Method

Use a fresh or frozen fruit of your choice. Combine fruit and lemon juice and cook, covered, about 20 minutes; stir often. Add softened gelatin and stir until dissolved. Fruits such as blueberries or boysenberries are nice when kept whole. Add sweetener after the jam has cooled.

WHIPPED COTTAGE CHEESE

20 calories
per tablespoon

Put low-fat cottage cheese in a blender and whip to a smooth consistency. Use as you would mayonnaise or sour cream.

LA COSTA SPA COCKTAIL SAUCE

Yields: 2 cups
10 calories per tablespoon

Ingredients

1 11-oz. bottle of dietetic
    ketchup (no sugar or salt)
1 Tbsp. freshly squeezed
    lemon juice

¼ cup freshly grated
    horseradish
¼ cup chopped chives
    (optional)

Method

Mix the first three ingredients in the order given. (Adjust horseradish and lemon to taste.) Refrigerate covered. Serve very cold or very hot. Add fresh chives just before serving if desired.

LA COSTA SPA COURT BOUILLON

Ingredients

1 cup dry white wine
4 cups water
1 onion
1 carrot

1 stalk celery
2 sprigs parsley
1 bay leaf
juice of 1 lemon strained

Method

Combine ingredients and simmer one-half hour. Strain the stock and use for poaching fish or shellfish.

DESSERTS

FRESH PINEAPPLE YOGURT

2 servings of
40 calories each

Ingredients

4 oz. low-fat yogurt (65–80 calories). Use nonfat yogurt if available (40 calories).

¼ cup coarsely chopped fresh pineapple

artificial sweetener (optional)
a few drops vanilla or lemon extract
dash cinnamon or nutmeg

Method

Combine yogurt with pineapple, sweetener, and flavorings to taste — or top the yogurt with fresh fruit only. (Handle yogurt with care because it tends to separate.) Put chilled yogurt into small sherbet glasses. Garnish just before serving with one teaspoon artificially sweetened fresh fruit or jam. Serve at once. Calorie count differs with the fruit used.

HOT APPLE COMPOTE

4 servings of
40 calories each

Ingredients

2 small golden delicious apples
½ cup unsweetened apple juice
1 cup water

1 stick cinnamon
2 orange slices, unpeeled

Method

Peel the apples and cut into quarters. Combine the apple juice, water, and cinnamon stick and simmer for about 2 minutes. Pour the hot juice over the apples; add the orange slices. Bake at 300° covered, for 10–20 minutes or until the apples can be pierced easily with a fork.

AMBROSIA

6 servings of
40 calories each

Ingredients

½ cup sliced fresh pineapple
½ cup diced papaya
½ cup diced mango
1 medium orange, peeled and
    sectioned

6 grapefruit sections
¼ cup plain low-fat yogurt
artificial sweetener to taste
1 drop red food coloring
    (optional)

Method

Combine the sliced fruits in a mixing bowl and arrange the fruit into individual serving dishes. Blend the yogurt, sweetener, and food coloring together. Top each serving of fruit with some of the yogurt mixture. Serve well chilled.

FROZEN BLUEBERRY YOGURT

8 servings of
40 calories each

Ingredients

1 cup frozen unsweetened
    blueberries
1 tsp. plain gelatin, dissolved
    in water

2 cups plain low-fat yogurt
1 tsp. liquid artificial sweetener

Method

Blend the berries and softened gelatin into the yogurt; add the sweetener. Pour into a shallow pan and place in the freezer. Whip the mixture every 15–20 minutes with a fork until frozen, to incorporate air and to reduce the size of the ice crystals. Serve in chilled sherbet dishes.

HOT SPICED RED PLUMS

4 servings of
40 calories each

Ingredients

8 dietetic canned plums, with
    juice
1 stick cinnamon

pinch allspice
pinch ground cinnamon
2 tsp. lemon juice

Method

Drain the plums, reserving the juice. Heat the plum juice, cinnamon stick, allspice, ground cinnamon, and lemon juice. Add the plums just before serving. Heat through.

❖❖❖❖❖❖❖❖❖❖❖❖❖❖❖❖❖❖❖❖❖❖❖❖❖❖❖❖❖

COUPE ST. JACQUES

6 servings of
40 calories each

Ingredients

½ tsp. plain gelatin
1 cup buttermilk
¾ cup nonfat milk
1½ tsp. vanilla
1 tsp. grated lemon rind
½ cup chopped pitted
 unsweetened cherries

artificial sweetener to taste
½ cup chopped combined
 watermelon, cantaloupe,
 and crenshaw melon

Method

Soften the gelatin in a few drops of water until it is completely dissolved; combine with the buttermilk, nonfat milk, and vanilla in a blender. Whip the mixture to a froth; add the lemon rind, cherries, and sweetener; blend again. Place the mixture in a shallow pan and freeze to a mushy consistency. Beat the sherbet with a wire whip or fork to get a lot of air into it and to keep the ice crystals very small. Keep whipping every 15–20 minutes until the sherbet is frozen. Scoop out the sherbet with an ice cream scoop. Garnish each serving with one tablespoon of the melon.

❖❖❖❖❖❖❖❖❖❖❖❖❖❖❖❖❖❖❖❖❖❖❖❖❖❖❖❖❖

PRUNE WHIP

6 servings of
40 calories each

Ingredients

6 oz. dietetic canned prunes,
 with juice
1 tsp. plain gelatin, softened
 in water

2 egg whites, stiffly beaten
1 tsp. lemon juice
¼ tsp. vanilla extract

Method

In a blender, purée the prunes with the juice they are packed in. Add the softened gelatin and blend again. Simmer the purée uncovered in a heavy skillet to reduce the mixture; cool slightly. Add lemon juice and vanilla. Gently fold the purée into the beaten egg whites. Portion the prune whip into small individual serving dishes and chill thoroughly.

BAKED APPLES

4 servings of
40 calories each

Ingredients

4 small baking apples
¼ cup unsweetened apple juice
1 cup water

1 tsp. cinnamon
1 small orange, sliced

Method

Preheat the oven to 350°. Core the apples and remove one-fourth of the top peel. Place in a shallow baking pan. Combine the juice, water, and cinnamon; pour over the apples. Arrange the orange slices around the apples to help flavor the liquid. Cover the pan with aluminum foil and bake about 20–30 minutes or until fork-tender.

WHIPPED BANANA PUDDING

8 servings of
40 calories each

Ingredients

2 cups plain low-fat yogurt
½ tsp. plain gelatin, softened
   in water
1 large ripe banana

1 tsp. liquid sweetener
½ tsp. grated lemon rind
   (optional)
8 drops yellow food coloring

Method

Blend all ingredients except yogurt in a blender until smooth. Fold in the yogurt. Pour into individual sherbet glasses. Chill well.

PINEAPPLE-APRICOT SHERBET

8 servings of
40 calories each

Ingredients

1 cup buttermilk
1½ cups nonfat milk
1 tsp. plain gelatin, softened
   in water
1 tsp. liquid sweetener
½ cup unsweetened canned
   pineapple chunks, drained

4 medium unsweetened
   apricot halves
2 Tbsp. vanilla extract
grated rind of 1 lemon
   or orange

Method

Blend all ingredients throughly. Place the mixture in a shallow pan and freeze until mushy. Whip with a fork to incorporate air. Repeat the whipping every 15–20 minutes until the sherbet is set.

❖❖❖❖❖❖❖❖❖❖❖❖❖❖❖❖❖❖❖❖❖❖❖❖❖❖❖

FROZEN BANANA ORANGE YOGURT

6 servings of
40 calories each

Ingredients

1 small, very ripe banana
1 small orange, sectioned (all
  membrane removed)
1 tsp. liquid sweetener

1 tsp. lime juice
1 tsp. plain gelatin, softened
  in water
1 cup plain low-fat yogurt

Method

Place all ingredients except the yogurt in a blender; mix well. Fold in the yogurt. Place in a shallow pan in the freezer. Beat with a wire whip or fork quite frequently while the mixture is freezing to keep the ice crystals small. Scoop the frozen yogurt into chilled champagne glasses and serve immediately.

❖❖❖❖❖❖❖❖❖❖❖❖❖❖❖❖❖❖❖❖❖❖❖❖❖❖

BUTTERMILK SHERBET

4 servings of
40 calories each

Ingredients

1 tsp. plain gelatin
1½ cups buttermilk
¾ cup nonfat milk
1 Tbsp. vanilla extract

grated rind of 1 lemon
liquid artificial sweetener
  to taste

Method

Add a few drops of cold water and two tablespoons boiling water to the gelatin; stir — over heat, if necessary — until gelatin is entirely dissolved. Combine buttermilk, nonfat milk, vanilla, softened gelatin, lemon rind, and a few drops of sweetener. Pour the mixture into a shallow pan (about 2 inches deep) and place in the freezer. Whip it occasionally with a wire whip so that it becomes mushy (this also adds air and makes it fluffier). Make sure the sherbet is sweetened enough, because you cannot add any more sweetener once it is frozen. Freeze it until it is just hard enough to form balls with an ice cream scoop. Serve in chilled sherbet dishes. Fresh berries or chopped fruit may be sprinkled on the sherbet if desired.

LEMON GELATIN

2 servings of
40 calories each

Ingredients

1 Tbsp. plain gelatin
3 cups of water
juice of 2 whole lemons

artificial sweetener to taste
grated lemon rind

Method

Soften the gelatin in a little of the water. Heat the remaining water with the lemon juice and the softened gelatin. Combine well. Add the sweetener. Chill the gelatin thoroughly. Garnish with grated lemon rind.

FROZEN STRAWBERRY YOGURT

4 servings of
40 calories each

Ingredients

1 cup sliced fresh strawberries
1 tsp. plain gelatin, softened in
   warm water

artificial sweetener to taste
1 cup plain low-fat yogurt

Method

Blend berries, softened gelatin, and sweetener. Fold into the yogurt. Pour the mixture into a shallow pan and place it in the freezer. Beat it with a fork quite frequently while it is freezing to incorporate air and also to reduce the size of the ice crystals. When it is frozen, but not too hard, it can be scooped out with an ice cream scoop and served in a sherbet glass.

APPLE JUICE FRAPPÉ

4 servings of
40 calories each

Ingredients

6 oz. unsweetened apple juice
1 medium golden delicious
   apple, chopped

1 tsp. lime juice
artificial sweetener to taste

Method

Combine all ingredients in a blender and blend well. Pour into a shallow pan and place in the freezer. When the juice begins to freeze around the edges, beat with a fork every 15 minutes until frozen. Serve in chilled sherbet glasses.

APRICOT PARFAIT

4 servings of
40 calories each

Ingredients

1½ tsp. plain gelatin
16 canned unsweetened apricot
    halves, with juice

artificial sweetener to taste
2 tsp. lime juice

Method

Soften the gelatin in a little cold water. Drain apricots, reserving all juice, and cut into small pieces. Measure the amount of juice and add water, if necessary, to measure 1½ cups of liquid total. Combine this liquid with the gelatin. Allow to set for 20 minutes. Combine the apricots, thickened juice, sweetener, and lime juice. Refrigerate until slightly thickened. Fill parfait glasses with the apricots and chill until ready to serve.

BOYSENBERRY PARFAIT

4 servings of
40 calories each

Ingredients

2 cup unsweetened frozen
    boysenberries
1½ tsp. plain gelatin

artificial sweetener to taste
1 tsp. lime juice

Method

Soften the gelatin in a little cold water. Thaw the boysenberries, retaining the juice. Measure the juice and add water if necessary to measure 1½ cups total. Combine the juice and gelatin. Allow to set for 20 minutes. Combine the berries, thickened juice, sweetener, and the lime juice. Refrigerate until slightly thickened. Fill parfait glasses with the berries and chill until ready to serve.

FRESH GRAPES

4 servings of
40 calories each

Ingredients

6 oz. fresh grapes

Method

Wash the grapes well and serve in chilled champagne glasses. The grapes can be frozen before serving.

PUMPKIN CUSTARD LA COSTA

6 servings of
40 calories each

Ingredients

5 egg whites
2 cups nonfat milk
liquid artificial sweetener to
    taste
½ tsp. vanilla extract

½ cup puréed pumpkin
¼ tsp. mace
¼ tsp. nutmeg
¼ tsp. cinnamon
¼ tsp. ground cloves

Method

Blend the egg whites and a small amount of the milk until just combined; do not overmix. Add the remaining milk, sweetener, vanilla, pumpkin, and spices. Blend just enough to combine the ingredients. Fill 6 warmed custard cups with the mixture, place them in a pan of hot water, and bake at 350° for 45 minutes, or until set.

COCONUT CUSTARD

6 servings of
40 calories each

Ingredients

5 egg whites
2 cups nonfat milk
liquid artificial sweetener to
    taste

½ tsp. vanilla extract
yellow food coloring (optional)
1 Tbsp. unsweetened coconut,
    toasted in the oven

Method

Blend the egg whites and the milk until just combined; do not overmix. Add the remaining milk, sweetener, vanilla, and a few drops of food coloring. Blend just enough to combine the ingredients. Fill 6 warmed custard cups with the mixture, place them in a pan of hot water, and bake at 350° for 45 minutes, or until set. Chill thoroughly. Just before serving, sprinkle with the toasted coconut.

FRESH PINEAPPLE WEDGE

4 servings of
40 calories each

Ingredients

1 medium-size pineapple

Method

Cut the top and bottom off the pineapple. Slice lengthwise into eight sections; remove the core. Loosen the pineapple flesh from the rind with a knife and cut horizontally into bite-size pieces. Leave the pineapple pieces in the shell. Chill well before serving.

♦♦♦♦♦♦♦♦♦♦♦♦♦♦♦♦♦♦♦♦♦♦♦♦♦♦♦♦♦♦♦♦♦♦♦♦♦♦

HOT BAKED FRESH PEARS

4 servings of
40 calories each

Ingredients

2 small Anjou pears
¼ cup unsweetened apple juice
1 cup water
1 stick cinnamon

3 whole cloves
Pinch nutmeg
juice of 1 lime (optional)
artificial sweetener (optional)

Method

Slice the pears in half lengthwise; do not peel. Remove the core and seeds. Place the pears cut side down in a shallow baking pan. Combine the remaining ingredients and pour over the pears. Cover the pan with foil and bake at 350° for 12 minutes or until the pears are barely tender. Remove from the oven and allow the pears to cool slightly in the liquid. Serve warm.

♦♦♦♦♦♦♦♦♦♦♦♦♦♦♦♦♦♦♦♦♦♦♦♦♦♦♦♦♦♦♦♦♦♦♦♦♦♦

HOT SPICED PEACHES

4 servings of
40 calories each

Ingredients

8 unsweetened canned peach
    halves
pinch allspice
1 clove

pinch nutmeg
1 stick cinnamon
artificial sweetener (optional)

Method

Drain the juice from the peaches and reserve. Combine the peach juice and remaining ingredients in a small saucepan and bring to a boil. Place the peaches in a shallow baking pan and pour the juice over them; bake covered at 300° until the juice is thick, approximately 15–20 minutes. Serve hot.

HOT APRICOT COMPOTE

4 servings of
40 calories each

Ingredients

16 sun-dried apricot halves   ground cloves
cinnamon

Method

Place the apricots in an ovenproof pan and cover with water. Soak overnight.
About 30 minutes before serving, add cinnamon and cloves to taste. Bake the
apricots in the liquid, covered, for 15–20 minutes in a 300° oven. Serve hot.

FROZEN PINEAPPLE SLICES

4 servings of
40 calories each

Ingredients

1 20-oz. can unsweetened
   pineapple slices (10
   slices)

Method

Punch two holes in the top of the can of pineapple; do not drain. Place the can
in the freezer, juice and all, and allow to freeze for 3–4 hours. When ready to
serve, open the can and push the pineapple slices out. Separate them with a
knife and serve. Two slices equals 40 calories.

CHOCOLATE MOUSSE

4 servings of
40 calories each

Ingredients

1 tsp. plain gelatin   3 egg whites
½ cup cold water   ½ cup shaved ice
1 package low-calorie
   chocolate pudding mix

Method

Dissolve the gelatin in the cold water, then add the pudding mix, blending
well. Simmer the mixture slowly, stirring constantly until it thickens. Let the
mixture cool to room temperature. Beat the egg whites until frothy and add the
shaved ice slowly while beating. Continue beating until the egg whites hold a
peak. Fold the egg whites gently into the pudding mix, combining well. Spoon
into sherbet glasses and chill.

INDEX

(Entries in bold indicate names of exercises. Page numbers in bold indicate a table.)

RECIPE INDEX